AUTOANTIBODIES AND CYTOKINES

Edited by **Wahid Ali Khan**

Autoantibodies and Cytokines

http://dx.doi.org/10.5772/intechopen.68834
Edited by Wahid Ali Khan

Contributors

Roberto Pontarolo, Vinicius Lins Ferreira, Helena Hiemisch Lobo Borba, Aline De Fátima Bonetti, Letícia Paula Leonart, Ana Daneva Markova, Marija Hadzi Lega, Ivo Kjaev, Elena Dzikova, Goran Dimitrov, Jadranka Georgievska, Gligor Tofoski, Jonathan Blackburn, Farhanah Aziz, Muneerah Smith, Kaushiki Kadam, Purvi Mande, Asmita Choudhury, Neval Yurttutan Uyar, Takemi Otsuki, Suni Lee, Hiroaki Hayashi, Naoko Kumagai-Takei, Hidenori Matsuzaki, Kei Yoshitome, Nagisa Sada, Masayasu Kusaka, Kozo Urakami, Yasumitsu Nishimura, Maria Kazimiera Maślińska, Brygida Kwiatkowska, Liping Yu, Zhiyuan Zhao, Yong Gu, Jeremy Cheng, Wahid Ali Khan, Mohd Wajid Ali Khan, Subuhi Sherwani, Mushtaq Ahmed Khan, Mohammed Suliman Almogbel

First published in London, United Kingdom, 2019 by IntechOpen
IntechOpen is the global imprint of INTECHOPEN LIMITED, registered in England and Wales, registration number: 11086078, The Shard, 25th floor, 32 London Bridge Street
London, SE19SG – United Kingdom
Printed in Croatia

British Library Cataloguing-in-Publication Data
A catalogue record for this book is available from the British Library

Additional hard copies can be obtained from orders@intechopen.com

Autoantibodies and Cytokines, Edited by Wahid Ali Khan
p. cm.
Print ISBN 978-1-78984-852-6
Online ISBN 978-1-78984-853-3

For EU product safety concerns:
IN TECH d.o.o., Prolaz Marije Krucifikse Kozulić 3, 51000 Rijeka, Croatia,
info@intechopen.com or visit our website at intechopen.com.

Meet the editor

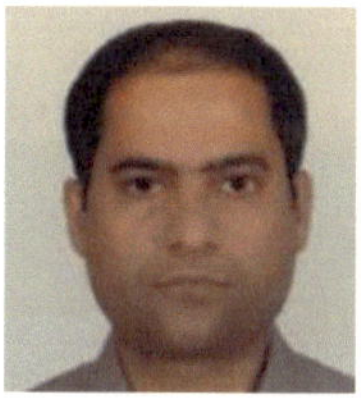

Dr. Wahid Ali Khan is an Assistant Professor in the Department of Clinical Biochemistry, College of Medicine, King Khalid University, Abha, KSA. Dr. Khan has served as a member of the editorial board of more than six international journals and has been guest editor for two journals. His research interests include the role of estrogen and its metabolites in various autoimmune diseases. He is also interested in cloning interferon alpha 2b and finding out its role in the pathogenesis of different types of autoimmune diseases. Dr. Khan has published more than 25 articles, 4 reviews, and 3 book chapters. He is also the editor of four books, which have been well recognized and documented by the international research community.

Contents

Preface

This book comes out with the idea that there is no complete resource that can explain autoantibodies and cytokines at the same time. These two molecules of immune system protect from the foreign bodies and are mainly responsible for various immunological processes. These molecules can function normally to give us defense and protect from foreign body. Somehow, slight changes in the body might trigger these molecules to act on their own cell and consider them alien. This may trigger various immune responses and protective antibodies are now acted on normal cells and tissues and presented them as foreign. At this time, they are called as "autoantibodies" and they trigger series of reactions that might escape from normal body's security check up. Other molecules of the immune system like cytokines remain helpless and they leave the idea that these autoantibodies are not doing anything wrong. As these molecules growing their function in negative prospective, so there might be a good chance to use them as diagnostic and prognostic marker for autoimmune diseases.

The order of the topic for this book follows general trends of the book, starting from the basic followed by their role in different diseases and their assay. This book has four sections: "Autoantibodies", "Cytokines and Interferons", "Autoantibodies and cytokines in different diseases" and "Autoantibodies based biomarker and their assay". The first section of the book includes three chapters that discuss general about autoantibodies, their structure, physiology and function as key mediators for autoimmune infertility. The first introductory chapter explains general about autoantibodies and their subtypes. Second chapter deals with the structure, physiology and function of autoantibodies. The third chapter explains autoantibodies as key mediators for autoimmune infertility.

Second section includes one chapter that explains the structures and functions of cytokines and interferon. In this section, chapter four deals with the function and types of cytokines and interferon.

Third section of the book " Autoantibodies and cytokines in different diseases" deals with the role of autoantibodies and cytokines in various autoimmune diseases and related complications. This section starts with the role of autoantibodies in viral diseases, followed by their role in autoimmune diseases, primary Sjogreen's syndrome and silicosis. This section also explains preeclampsia in relation to the cytokines in pregnancy.

Fourth section "Autoantibodies based biomarker and their assay" consists of two chapters that deal with the usage of autoantibodies as biomarker in disease staging, treatment motoring and contemporary technological approaches to autoantibodies biomarker discovery and validity, and finally, their assays in autoimmune disease. Overall, this book is a collection of latest topic on autoantibodies and cytokines that guide those who seeks to improve their knowledge for this topic.

Dr. Wahid Ali Khan
Assistant Professor
Clinical Biochemistry
College of Medicine
King Khalid University
Abha, KSA

Section 1

Autoantibodies

Chapter 1

Introductory Chapter: Autoantibodies and Their Types

Wahid Ali Khan

Additional information is available at the end of the chapter

http://dx.doi.org/10.5772/intechopen.77328

1. Introduction

Autoantibodies are groups of antibodies that are directed against body's own antigen. These autoantibodies are generated against different types of antigens in various autoimmune diseases. Clinical symptoms of systemic autoimmune diseases are characterized by the involvement of various organs in addition to the production of non-organ specific autoantibodies. These autoantibodies in autoimmune diseases are associated with a specific clinical symptom within a spectrum [1]. Most of the autoantibodies have diagnostic and prognostic importance with respect to their associated disease and all of these are not involve in the pathogenesis of these diseases. Most autoantibodies are mainly used as biological markers for certain disease but they do not actually reflect the pathophysiological process underwent during the course of the disease, **however, many autoantibodies also have a pathogenetic roles such as anti-nuclear antibodies and anti-tTG antibodies in celiac disease**. For example, autoimmune hepatitis is a chronic disease which is characterized by various clinical, histological as well as immunological characteristics including production of circulating autoantibodies and high serum concentration of gamma globulin [2]. These autoantibodies are very important for the correct diagnosis and classification of autoimmune liver disease [3] and they are not related with the pathogenesis of autoimmune hepatitis. However, some of the systemic autoimmune disease relating these autoantibodies in the sense that their levels are changes during the course of the disease. These include anti-double stranded DNA antibodies in systemic lupus erythematosus (SLE) and anti-neutrophil cytoplasmic autoantibodies in the vasculitis [4]. Other types of antibodies like anti-nucleosome and anti-CIq autoantibodies can function as both markers of the disease activity as well as pathogenic autoantibodies in SLE [5, 6].

The history of the autoantibodies goes back to 1940s, when two types of antibodies (anti-nuclear antibodies; ANA and rheumatoid factors; RF) were discovered as the serum factors that bind to nuclear antigen IgG, respectively [7, 8]. ANA and RF considered being a diagnostic feature of SLE but their role in disease pathogenesis remains elusive. In the last two decades, the effects of autoimmune diseases have been gown up to such an extent that it can explains both points of views, as clinically and diagnostically. The pathogenic mechanisms of these autoimmune diseases help to contribute to the discovery of new autoantibodies and new area of research, based on diagnostic and prognostic value, have been developed. Determination of these autoantibodies in the diagnosis of autoimmune disease is important because they are sometime showing nonspecific, unclear character and even shared by different autoimmune diseases [9]. For most of the autoimmune diseases, classification criteria include the determination of autoantibody that helps in final diagnosis. They are important not only for diagnostic perspective but also for prognostic value. Some of these autoimmune have been associated with the clinical manifestation of the disease, therefore estimation of these autoantibodies pattern in the patients might helpful to detect severity of the disease that can be useful for the need of correct therapy [10].

Several autoimmune diseases show chronic conditions that develop over the period of years and are characterized by the production of autoantibodies that actually present much before the actual onset of the disease. These autoantibodies are called as predictive autoantibodies that are present (or appear) in the blood much before systemic pathological conditions arise during the course of the disease. Detection of specific autoantibodies is the most important clinical and experimental evidence to predict any autoantibodies as biomarker for that autoimmune disease [11]. The levels and variety of autoantibodies may vary according to the disease that may function as predictive biomarker. While the experimental importance of autoantibodies has been well recognized in many clinical conditions, its clinical utilization remains to be short for most of the diseases [12]. Autoimmune diseases are caused by various autoimmune responses, generated during the course of the disease. The generations of immune responses are characterized by the appearance of the autoantibodies in the serum, therefore recognition of a particular autoantibody showed the path to recognize an autoimmune disease. Initially, the clinical symptoms of the disease are not emerges in full flash although these autoantibodies may arises much before these symptoms and actual onset of the disease. So, the symptoms are not visible, so the physician did not think to test these autoantibodies initially [13]. Therefore, test for these autoantibodies could be done in pre-screening on various groups of population to identify the individuals who are susceptible for the development of the disease at an early stages and treatment should be given to prevent the actual occurrence of the disease. Multiple tests have been given for these patients for different autoimmune diseases, and recommendations are given to done multiple test for the patient who are having autoimmune disease [14]. However, disease related autoantibodies cannot develop simultaneously, although they are present much before the actual disease onset, and many of these autoantibodies are antigen specific, so using a panel of different autoantibodies set, might helpful to increase the sensitivity and prediction of the test [15].

Autoimmunity arises due to the failure of the immune system to be self-tolerance, which is mediated through the involvement of T and B cells [16]. Most of the autoimmune disease involves T cell, which play an important role in dysregulation and autoimmune aggression and during this process large amount of autoantibodies are also produced. These autoantibodies plays not only in key pathogenic role in some diseases including SLE and Graves' disease but also found in some disease in which they play minor pathogenic role and can act as important biomarker [17, 18]. Cytokines, in addition to the production of autoantibodies, play important role in the generation of autoimmune response (especially pro-inflammatory cytokines: except multiple sclerosis), they are produced in response to the viral invasion and are deeply involved in various autoimmune process. Under normal condition, anti-cytokine antibodies response have been develop in healthy normal individual that is consider to be normal physiological process to control various immune response. These responses are for limited time initially, and then the concentration of these autoantibodies increases, reaching a threshold and then coming up to its normal concentration after few weeks. This process also occurs in some pathological conditions including autoimmunity and autoantibodies develop as a result of these processes might be used as prognostic marker for monitoring the disease [19].

2. Different types of autoantibodies

2.1. Anti-cytokine autoantibodies

Autoantibodies against various types of cytokines have been described not only in normal individuals but also in patients with different infectious and immuno-inflammatory disease [20]. These include interferon (α, β, and γ), interleukin (α, 2, 4, 6, 8 and 10), nerve growth factor, chemokine (α and β), leukemia inhibitory factor, granulocyte-macrophage colony-stimulating factor, and tumor necrosis factor (α and β) and receptor, which are found to be in normal individuals and patients with various disorders. In autoimmune disease, these autoantibodies can function as prognostic biomarkers that may even show negative (autoantibodies against IL-18 and IL-1α in RA) or positive (autoantibodies to IL-6 in systemic sclerosis) results [21]. The autoantibodies against cytokines found to be pathogenic that makes autoimmune patients more susceptible to other diseases. There are various autoimmune diseases including rheumatoid arthritis, multiple sclerosis, systemic sclerosis, SLE, autoimmune polyendocrine syndrome type 1, in which neutralizing autoantibodies against cytokines have been described. The affinity of anti-cytokine autoantibodies may depend on the function of cytokine during various immune responses. For example, pro-inflammatory cytokines such as interleukin-1α, -6, -8, TNF-α and GM-CSF, have more frequently autoantibodies, whereas anti-inflammatory cytokines like interleukin-10 and TGF-β, have autoantibodies that were reported rarely [22–24]. However, most of these studies does not provide sufficient evidences for the functional effects of these autoantibodies, which might helpful to describe their role in various autoimmune diseases and capitalize them for future therapies. There are few pro-inflammatory cytokines that play important role in joint aggression in rheumatoid arthritis [25, 26]. Autoantibodies against IL-1alpha can be worked as an important prognostic marker for early detection of RA [27] and several parameters of RA disease activity and severity was found to be significantly lower in those patients who have high levels of anti-IL-1α autoantibodies in comparison to those who have low levels of these autoantibodies. Autoantibodies showed neutralizing effects on the function of IL-1α by inhibiting thymocytes proliferation in the sera of RA patients [28]. These autoantibodies were also detected in the patients with systemic sclerosis. Autoantibodies against IL-1α have been secreted in high amount in the skin [29]. These autoantibodies have also been found in other dermal diseases; for example, psoriasis and pemphigus, that are supposed to be involve in the regulation of inflammation of skin [30].

2.2. Antinuclear autoantibodies (ANA)

Autoimmune hepatitis is the first disease in which autoantibodies had been clearly associated. In 1960s, these autoantibodies were detected by indirect immunofluorescence assay in the diagnosis and prognosis of autoimmune hepatitis. ANA directed against various nuclear components including single or double stranded DNA (s- or ds-DNA), transfer RNA, histone and other nuclear components [31–33]. There are various other nuclear components which are targeted by these autoantibodies but are not related with autoimmune hepatitis including s-DNA and ds-DNA, chromatin, histones, hnRNP, A_2/B_1, cyclin A, and centromere of the chromosomes [34]. These autoantibodies may arise due to the mistake in identifying normal nuclear components as foreign and dangerous. Once this happen, they identify natural occurring protein as foreign and they are called as autoantibodies because they are produce against own antigen. These autoantibodies start chains of reactions causing inflammation and attack itself. So they also start to target normal protein in the nucleus of the cell and they are called antinuclear antibodies. Although, we all have autoantibodies but they are present in very small amount and they remain silent in the body until and unless some factors may trigger these autoantibodies to be active against normal nuclear components. Once these autoantibodies attack on the self nuclear components, they may trigger various diseases including systemic lupus erythematosus, scleroderma, Sjogren's syndrome, polymyositis/dermatomyositis, etc. Increased level of ANA is seen in almost all the systemic rheumatic disease which either showed sometime high, sometime loose association between a particular type of ANA and a particular type of rheumatic disease. Most of these autoantibodies directed against either nucleic acids or protein close to the nucleic acid. For example, the most common antigen in SLE is nucleosomes. Nucleosomes form the building blocks of chromatin molecule and play an important role in the compaction of DNA in the nucleus. ANA directed against DNA, considered to be as diagnostic maker and hallmark of SLE. Antibodies against histones were also reported in various studies that also proven to be an important marker for SLE. Other important antigen for ANA is small nuclear ribonucleoprotein (snRNP) particles that are formed from a capped small nuclear RNA molecule and polypeptide. In addition, other antigens from the cytoplasmic relevance to ANA binding are ribosomal RNP and aminoacyl tRNA synthetase [35]. ANA play an active role in SLE since these autoantibodies bind to the antigen that may be present in the circulation or their immune complexes are deposited in the tissue that leads to inflammation and subsequent disease features. Either anti-DNA or anti-DNA complexes were involved in the induction of lupus nephritis. In addition, anti-DNA antibodies against various protein molecules are also found in SLE that plays an important role in the etiopathogenesis of this disease [36–40].

2.3. Anti-citrullinated protein antibodies and anti-CCP antibodies

These are the autoantibodies that are induced against any peptide or protein that are citrullinated. They are present in the majority of the patients suffering from RA. Clinically, this antigen can be frequently used to detect antibodies in the serum of RA patients. It has been assumed that high titers of these autoantibodies are correlated with high risk in the development of RA [41]. These autoantibodies were found to be highly sensitive and specific in comparison to rheumatoid factor. In addition, combined estimation of rheumatoid factor and anti-citrulline antibodies can increase the assessment of both tests [41]. Anti-CCP antibodies can function not only as diagnostic marker but also have prognostic value, they might be used to predict the development of the disease and can be present much before the actual onset of the disease. These autoantibodies are also associated with other diseases such as cardiovascular as well as pulmonary complications. Anti-CCP antibodies can be useful in the diagnosis and prognosis of RA and have been included as one of the major criteria for the classification of this disease [42].

2.4. Rheumatoid factor (RF)

Rheumatoid arthritis is one of the disease in which the option for diagnosis and prognosis is more advance in the field of autoimmunity [43]. Since RA have nonspecific symptoms, therefore the diagnosis could be difficult but early diagnosis is important to have more option for therapy and cure. However, as this disease is characterized by radiological progression during early phase of the disease, so there might be good opportunity to initiate for early and effective treatment [44]. In early studies, serological diagnostic tool for RA were limited and the only autoantibodies related with the diagnosis of RA was rheumatoid factor that showed low sensitivity and specificity [43, 44]. Some patients can even showed negativity for RF and RF may be positive in various other autoimmune diseases that are showing nonclinical conditions and are positive even with other types of autoantibodies in these diseases. If the RF is falsely positive, it is interesting to mention that the complementary diagnostic test is antistreotolysin O (ASO/ASLO) test. Earlier studies have shown that smoker have elevated incidence of RA because of high RF [45]. Studies also indicated that elevated level of RF was found to be twice in comparison to both current and ex-smokers than nonsmokers and the level of RF was more in these individual [46]. Studies also have shown that smoking somehow effect the progression of RA [47].

Besides that, there are large groups of autoantibodies that are causing various types of autoimmune diseases including Anti-transglutaminase antibodies-celiac disease, dermatitis herpetiformis; Anti-ganglioside antibodies-Miller-Fisher syndrome, acute motor axonal neuropathy; Anti-actin antibodies-coeliac disease; Anti-thrombin antibodies-SLE; Anti-neutrophil cytoplasmic antibody-polyangiitis; Anti-smooth muscles antibodies-hepatitis; Anti-mitochondrial antibodies-primary biliary cirrhosis; Anti-SRP-polymyositis; Anti-SRP & Anti-AChR-myasthenia gravis; Anti-thyroid antibodies-Hashimoto's thyroiditis, Graves' disease; Anti-SLA/LP, perinuclear anti-cytoplasmic antibodies, Anti-LKM, Anti-LC-1, Anti-mitochondrial antibodies, Anti-asialoglycoprotein receptor antibodies-liver disease, etc. (**Figure 1**).

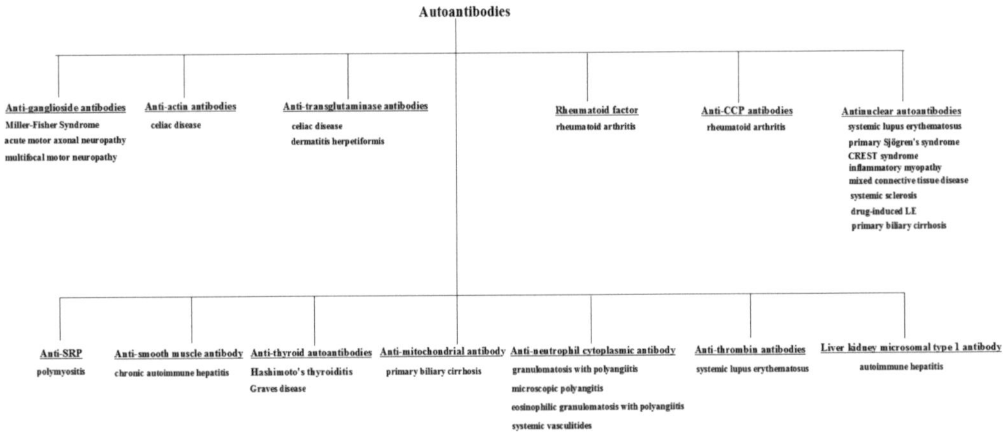

Figure 1. List of some common autoantibodies and their associated diseases.

3. Conclusion

Autoantibodies are group of antibodies that are directed against self antigen. These antibodies recognized normal molecules in the cells as foreign and dangerous. As a result of that, large group of reactions take place in which these autoantibodies recognized normal molecules and generate various immunological response against them. In consequence, these autoantibodies also interact with other protein molecule in order to generate a series of reactions causing binding to the self molecules. Binding of autoantibodies to self molecules can be recognized by various immune cells that mainly responsible for the damage and excretion of these molecules. For examples, there are various types of autoantibodies and their associated antigens found in in SLE (**Table 1**). These self damaged molecules are called as auto-antigen and finally treat as foreign molecule and damage by various immune cells.

Antinuclear autoantibodies (ANA)	Various nuclear components
Anti-ds DNA	Double stranded DNA
Anti-Sm	Protein with nuclear U1 RNA
Anti-RNP	Protein with U1 RNAγ
Anti-R_o (SS-A)	Protein with hYRNA
Anti-La (SS-B)	Protein with hYRNA
Anti-histone	Histones
Anti-phospholipids	Phospholipids
Anti-neuronal	Neurons and lymphocytes
Anti-ribosomal	Protein in ribosomes

Table 1. Major types of autoantibodies and their associated antigens in SLE.

http://dx.doi.org/10.5772/intechopen.77328

Author details

Wahid Ali Khan

Address all correspondence to: wahidalikhan@rediffmail.com

Clinical Biochemistry, College of Medicine, King Khalid University, Abha, KSA

References

[1] Wiik AS. Anti-nuclear autoantibodies: Clinical utility for diagnosis, prognosis, monitoring and planning of treatment strategy in systemic immunoinflammatory disease. Scandinavian Journal of Rheumatology. 2005;**34**:260-268

[2] Manus MP, Czaja AJ, Gorham JD, Krawitt EL, Micli-Vergani G, Vergani D, et al. Diagnosis and management of autoimmune hepatitis. Hepatology. 2010;**51**:2193-2213

[3] Sener AG. Autoantibodies in autoimmune liver diseases. APMIS. 2015;**123**:915-919

[4] Kallenberg CGM, Stegeman CA, Bootsma H, Bijl M, Limburg PC. Quantitation of autoantibodies in systemic autoimmune disease: Clinically usefull? Lupus. 2006;**15**:397-402

[5] Amoura Z, Koutouzov S, Chabre H, et al. Presence of antinucleosome autoantibodies in a restricted set of connective tissue disease: Antinucleosome antibodies of the IgG 3 subclass are markers of renal oathogenicity in systemic lupus erythematosus. Arthritis and Rheumatism. 2000;**43**:76-84

[6] Trouw LA, Groeneveld TW, Seelen MA, et al. Anti-CIq autoantibodies deposit in glomeruli but are only pathogenic in combination with glomeruli C1q-cintaing immune complexes. The Journal of Clinical Investigation. 2004;**114**:679-688

[7] Robbin WC, Holman HR, Deicher H, Kunkel HG. Complement fixation with cell nuclear and DNA in lupus erythematosus. Proceedings of the Society for Experimental Biology and Medicine. 1957;**96**:575-579

[8] Miescher P, Fauconnet M. Absorption of L.E. factor by isolated cell nuclei. Experientia: Interdisciplinary Journal for the Life Sciences. 1954;**10**:252-253

[9] Stinton LM, Fritzler MJ. Clinical approach of autoantibody testing in systemic autoimmune rheumatic disease. Autoimmunity Reviews. 2007;**7**:77-84

[10] Avouac J, Gossec L, Dougados M. Diagnostic and predictive value of anti-cyclic citrullinated protein antibodies in rheumatoid arthritis: A systemic literature review. Annals of the Rheumatic Diseases. 2006;**65**:845-851

[11] Bizzaro N. Autoantibodies as predictors of disease: The clinical and experimental evidence. Autoimmunity Reviews. 2007;**6**:325-333

[12] Lernmark A. Autoimmune disease: Are markers ready for prediction? The Journal of Clinical Investigation. 2001;**108**:1091-1096

[13] Rose NR. Prediction and prevention of autoimmune disease: A personal perspective. Annals of the New York Academy of Sciences. 2007;**1109**:117-128

[14] Tonutti E, Visentini D, Bizaro N. Interpretative comments on autoantibodies tests. Autoimmunity Reviews. 2007;**6**:341-346

[15] Bizzaro N. The predictive significance of autoantibodies in organ-specific autoimmune disease. Clinical Reviews in Allergy and Immunology. 2007;**34**:326-331

[16] Kearney JF. Formation of autoantibodies, including anti-cytokine antibodies is a hallmark of the immune response of early B cells. Journal of Interferon Research. 1994;**14**:151-152

[17] Ozen S, Berk O, Simsek DG, Darcans S. Clinical cause of Hashimoto's thyroiditis and effects of levothyroxine therapy on the clinical course of the disease in children and adolescents. Journal of Clinical Research in Pediatric Endocrinology. 2011;**3**:192-197

[18] McKee A, Peyer F. TSI assay utilization: Impact on costs of graves hyperthyroidism diagnosis. The American Journal of Managed Care. 2012;**18**:e1-e14

[19] Graudal NA, Svenson M, Trap U, Garred P, et al. Autoantibodies against interleukin 1 alpha in rheumatoid arthritis: Association with long term radiographic outcome. Annals of the Rheumatic Diseases. 2002;**61**:598-602

[20] Bendtzen K, Hansen MB, Ross C, Svenson M. Detection of autoantibodies to cytokines. Molecular Biotechnology. 2000;**14**:251-261

[21] Cappellano G, Orilieri E, Woldetsadik AD, et al. Anti-cytokine autoantibodies in autoimmune disease. American Journal of Clinical and Experimental Immunology. 2012;**1**:136-146

[22] Svenson M, Poulsen LK, Fomsgaard A, Bendtzen K. IgG autoantibodies against interleukin 1 alpha in sera of normal individual. Scandinavian Journal of Immunologyl. 1989;**29**:489-492

[23] Hansen MB, Svenson M, Diamant M, Bendtzen K. Anti-interleukin-6 antibodies in normal human serum. Scandinavian Journal of Immunology. 1991;**33**:777-781

[24] Elkarim RA, Mustafa M, Kivisak P, et al. Cytokine autoantibodies in multiple sclerosis, aseptic meningitis and stroke. European Journal of Clinical Investigation. 1998;**28**:295-299

[25] Arend WF, Dayer JM. Inhibition of the production and effects of interleukin-1 and tumor necrosis factor a in rheumatoid arthritis. Arthritis and Rheumatism. 1995;**38**:151-160

[26] Le Huu D, Matsushita T, Jin G, et al. IL-6 blockade attenuates the development of Murin sclerodermatous chronic graft-versus-host disease. The Journal of Investigative Dermatology. 2012;**132**:2752-2761

[27] Jouvenne P, Fossiez F, Banchereau J, Miossec P. High levels of neutralizing autoantibodies against IL-1alpha are associated with a better prognosisi in chronic polyarthritis: A follow-up study. Scandinavian Journal of Immunology. 1997;**46**:413-418

[28] Suzuki H, Kamimura J, Ayabe T, Kashiwagi H. Demosntration of neutralizing autoantibodies ahainst IL-1alpha in cera from patients with rheumatoid arthritis. Journal of Immunology. 1990;**145**:2140-2146

[29] Jouvenne P, Fossiez F, Garroue P, et al. Increased incidence of neutralizing autoantibodies against interleukin-1alpha (IL-1alpha) in nondestructive chronic polyarthritis. Journal of Clinical Immunology. 1996;**16**:283-290

[30] Mizutani H, Ohmoto Y, Kupper TS, Shimizu M. Endogenous neutralizing anti-IL-1alpha autoantibodies in inflammatory skin disease: Possible natural inhibitor for over expressed epidermal IL-1. Journal of Dermatological Science. 1998;**20**:63-71

[31] Bagdanos DP, Chaudhari K, Vergani D. Molecule mimicry and autoimmune liver disease: virtuous intensions, malign consequence. Liver. 2001;**21**:225-232

[32] Hennes EM, Zeniya M, Aj C, et al. Simplified criteria for the diagnosis of autoimmune hepatitis. Hepatology. 2008;**48**:169-176

[33] Strassburg CP, Manns MP. Autoantibodies and autoantigens in autoimmune hepatitis. Seminars in Liver Disease. 2002;**22**:339e52

[34] Johanet C, Beleoken E, Ballot E. Autoantibodies in autoimmune hepatitis: Antinuclear antibodies (ANA). Clinics and Research in Hepatology and Gastroenterology. 2012;**36**: 394-396

[35] Smeenk RJI, Feltkamp TEW. Antinuclear antibodies. In: Delves PJ, Roitt I, editors. Encyclopedia of Immunology. London: Academic Press; 1998. pp. 125-133

[36] Khan WA, Qureshi JA. Increased binding of circulating systemic lupus erythematosus autoantibodies to recombinant interferon alpha 2b. APMIS. 2015;**123**:1016-1024

[37] Khan WA, Moinuddin, Habib S. Preferential recognition of catecholestrogen modified DNA by circulating autoantibodies in cancer patients. Biochemie. 2013;**95**:329-335

[38] Khan WA, Moinuddin Khan MWA, Chabbra HS. Catecholestrogen: Possible role in systemic lupus erythematosus. Rheumatology. 2009;**48**:1345-1351

[39] Khan WA, Habib S, Khan MWA, Alam K. Moinuddin. Enhanced binding of circulating SLE autoantibodies to catecholestrogen-copper-modified DNA. Molecular and Cellular Biochemistry. 2008;**315**:143-150

[40] Khan WA. Binding characteristics of SLE anti-DNA autoantibodies to catechol-estrogen modified DNA. Scandinavian Journal of Immunology. 2006;**64**:667-683

[41] van der Linden MPM, van der Woude D, Ioan-Facsinary A, et al. Value of anti-modified citrullinated vimentin and third generation anti-cyclic citrullinated peptide compared with second generation anti-cyclic citrullinated peptide and rheumatoid factor in predicting disease outcome in undifferentiated arthritis and rheumatoid arthritis. Arthritis and Rheumatism. 2009;**60**:2232-2241

[42] Gerosa M. Autoantibodies and autoimmune disease: An update. Clinics in Dermatology. 2013;**2**:72-76

[43] de Rooy DP, van der Linden MP, Knevel R, et al. Predicting arthritis outcomes-what can be learned from the Leiden early arthritis clinic? Rheumatology. 2011;**50**:93-100

[44] vander Woude D, Young A, Vayakumar K, et al. Prevalence of and predictive factors for sustained disease-modifying antirheumatic drug-free remission in rheumatoid arthritis. Results from two large early arthritis cohorts. Arthritis and Rheumatism. 2009;**60**:2262-2271

[45] Jonsson T, Thoosteinsson J, Valdimarsson H. Does smoking stimulate rheumatoid factor production in rheumatic individuals. APMIS. 1998;**106**:970-974

[46] Heliovaara M, Aho K, Aromaa A, et al. Smoking and risk of rheumatoid arthritis. The Journal of Rheumatology. 1993;**20**:1830-1835

[47] Saaq KG, Cerhan JR, Kolluri S, et al. Cigarette smoking and rheumatoid arthritis severity. Annals of the Rheumatic Diseases. 1997;**56**:463-469

Chapter 2

Structure, Physiology, and Functions of Autoantibodies

Neval Yurttutan Uyar

Additional information is available at the end of the chapter

http://dx.doi.org/10.5772/intechopen.76020

Abstract

Prevalence of autoimmune diseases is increasing. Antibodies are responsible for the humoral type of adaptive immune responses, glycoprotein structure and produced by B lymphocytes. Failure of Immunologic self-tolerance due to environmental and genetic factors may predipose the development of autoimmunity. Self-antigens are either tolerogenic or ignored. Central tolerance occurs at immature T and B lymphocytes in the thymus and bone marrow. Peripheral tolerance occurs at mature lymphocytes encounter self-antigens in peripheral tissues. Negative selection, regulatory T cells, anergy, activation-induced cell death, immune suppression, receptor editing are examples of important steps of immune tolerance. B lymphocytes that produce antibodies which bind self-antigen with medium/low affinity escape from anergy and those antibodies are called as natural autoantibodies but the other ones with high affinity are undergo anergy, The natural antibodies have play critical roles as; discrimination foreign from self, auto-multireactivity, regulate the immunomodulation, maintain tissue homeostasis. Natural autoantibodies work as the templates for the production of pathogenic autoantibodies which has high affinity, switch the class and diverse somatically under proper conditions. Pathogenic autoantibodies can protect or cause diseases via neutralization of self-antigens, opsonization, antibody-dependent cellular cytotoxicity, activation of the complement system, pro-inflammatory and anti-inflammatory effect.

Keywords: physiology, function, structure, autoantibody

1. Introduction

Autoimmune diseases have been increased for the past decades worldwide [1, 2].The prevalence of autoantibodies induced autoimmune diseases is over 2.5% [3].

Failure of immunologic tolerance may cause the development of autoimmune response and then autoimmune disease [4, 5].

The cause of autoimmune diseases is an association of genetic tendency and environmental factors cause alteration the immune regulatory genes by diver's mechanisms as epigenetics. In autoimmune diseases pathogenesis, both cellular (as in multiple sclerosis) and humoral (as in systemic lupus erythematosus (SLE)) type of the adaptive immune system takes a role. An autoimmune response does not inevitably signify the autoimmune disease [5, 6].

In most of autoimmune diseases, the autoantibodies could been found but not all. Even in some autoimmune diseases, the autoantibodies signify not autoimmune disease risk, but also the level of the autoantibodies signifies the severity. By autoantibodies, we can understand immunologic tolerance failure and pathogenesis mechanisms [7–15].

Autoantibodies are self-reactive antibodies. The self-antigens may be found in all cell types (e.g. chromatin, centromeres) and those autoimmune diseases is systemic or be highly specific for a specific cell type in one organ of the body (e.g. thyroglobulin in cells of the thyroid gland) and those autoimmune diseases is organ-specific. The self-antigens can be in proteins, nucleic acids, carbohydrates, lipids structure [16]. Immune tolerance is succeed by various mechanisms, occurred at both central and peripheral organs.

2. Autoantibody structure

An antibody molecule and also autoantibody are include of four polypeptide chains; composed of a pair of identical *heavy* (H) and *light* (L) chains. Molecular weight of light chain is 25 kDa and heavy chain is 50–70 kDa. The four chains joint together as a Y shaped. Each light chain is bound to one heavy chain, and the two heavy chains are bound to each other by disulfide bonds between two cysteine amino acid.

The antigen-binding site of chains that diverse at different antibody is called as the *variable* (V) regions and composed of amino acid N-terminal domains of the heavy and light chains. The part next to the V region is called the *constant* (C) region. A light chain is made up of one V and one C region, and a heavy chain has one V and three (at IgG, IgA) or four (at IgM, IgE) C regions. Each of them is 110 amino acids in length and fields into a characteristic three-dimensional shape called immunoglobulin (Ig). There are three hypervariable regions or CDRs at each variable region of the heavy chain (VH) and of the light chain (VL) which is just 6–10 amino acids in length. CDR3 is the greatest variability of three hypervariable region, at the junction of the V and C regions [4, 5] **Figure 1**.

Fab fragment (fragment antigen binding) is composed of a bonded whole light chain (with one V and one C region) and a heavy chain's V and first C region and recognizes the antigen. The Fc fragment (fragment crystalline) is the remaining region of heavy chain. Each antibody

http://dx.doi.org/10.5772/intechopen.76020

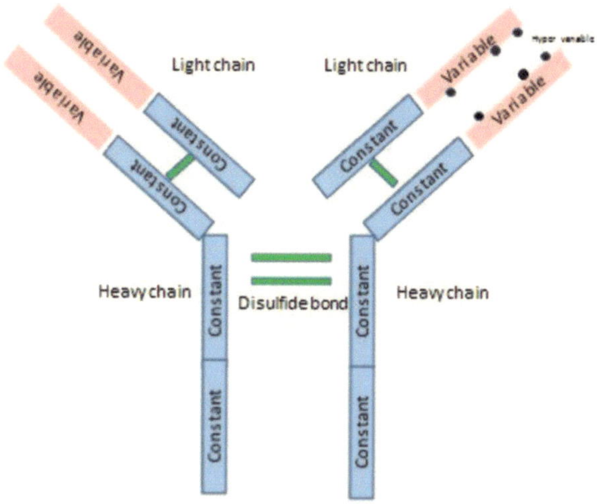

Figure 1. Structure of an antibody molecule (IgG).

contains two identical Fab fragments and one Fc fragment. The hinge region is located in the middle of the Fab and Fc regions and is very bending so helps the two Fab fragment getting closer to antigen far away. The C-Terminal end of the heavy chain of bound antibodies can terminate with or without anchoring in the cell membrane, but the C-Terminal end of the light chain terminates freely without attaching the cell membrane [4, 5].

There are two types of light chains according to C region, called κ and λ. Their functions are same. 60% of antibodies are κ chains and 40% are λ chains There are five types of heavy chains also according to C region, called μ, δ, γ, ε and α. Every combination of heavy chain and light chain is available. Antibodies are classified and entitled according to their heavy chains types (IgM, IgD, IgG, IgE and IgA) [4, 5].

There is five antibody isotypes with different functions and physical and biological properties, summarized in **Table 1**.

1. IgM: Heavy chain type is μ. It has pentamere structure with five Fc fragments where complement binds. The antigen+ pentamere antibody+ complement bound to five Fc complex starts strong complement activation and is removed by phagocytic cells or complement mediated lysis. So IgM plays critical role in neutralization but it has relatively low affinity and cannot penetrate into cells/tissues because of the pentamere structure. Half-life of IgG is approximately 10 days [4, 5].

2. IgG: Heavy chain type is γ. It has monomere structure and penetration rate is high e.g. penetare through the placenta There are four classes of IgG: G1, G2, G3 and G4. 65% of total IgG is G1. G1 and G3 activate complement system if the antigen is protein structure and the protein antigens are removed by phagocytic cells. G2 and G4 play role if the antigen is

Property	IgM	IgG	IgA	IgD	IgE
Heavy chain type	μ	γ	α	δ	E
% of total immunglobulin in serum	9	75	15	0.2	0.004
Structure	Monomer or pentamer	Monomer	Monomer or dimer	Monomer	Monomer
Molecular weight (×1000)	900	150	170 or 400	180	190
Complement fixation	++	++	−	−	−
Cross the placenta	−	++	−	−	−
Allergic response	−	−	−	−	++
Antigen receptor at B cell	++	−	−	+	−
Secretoral response	−	−	++	−	−

Table 1. Physical, biological properties and functions of immunoglobulins.

carbohydrate structure. Half-life of IgG is approximately 21 days. Since IgG has high affinity and high molar concentrations in plasma, it makes neutralization [4, 5, 17]. It also makes opsonization because of γ receptors of phagocytes. If N-terminal end is N-acetyl glucosamine, the IgG act as pro-inflammatory and if there is sialic acid then act as anti-inflammatory.

3. IgA: Heavy chain type is α. It has monomere or mostly dimere structure which consists of two basic units joined by a J chain. There are two classes of IgA: A1 and A2. IgA1 is in the serum while IgA2 is in secretions as; colostrum, salivary, eye tear, respiratory, digestion and genital and make neutralization of antigens at the mucosal sites. A2; secretory IgA (sIgA) is protected from lytic enzymes in the digestion tract by secretory component (SC) which is a part of the receptor and remains attached to the IgA-dimer [4, 5, 17].

4. IgD: Heavy chain type is δ. It has monomere structure. There are two classes of IgD: soluble and bound IgD. While function in immunology of soluble IgD is not known yet, IgD that bound on the cell membrane of newly produced B lymphocytes with IgM, activates of newly produced B lymphocytes by antigens [4, 5, 17].

5. IgE: Heavy chain type is ε. It has monomere structure. IgE plays role in parasitic infections and allergic reactions by binding to specific IgE receptors on mast cells and basophiles [4, 5].

3. Physiology of autoantibody

3.1. Physiology of antibody

Antibodies are responsible for the humoral type of adaptive immune responses, glycoprotein structure and produced by B lymphocytes.

Antigens can directly bind to antigen receptors of specific B lymphocytes. The type of reversible bond is non-covalent as; electrostatic attraction, hydrogen bonds, Van der Waals-, charge interactions and hydrophobic forces. Membrane–bound antibodies (IgM and IgD type) work

http://dx.doi.org/10.5772/intechopen.76020

as antigen receptors of B lymphocytes (BLR) and can bind to antigens in proteins, lipids, carbohydrates and nucleic acids structures. T lymphocytes can react antigens just in protein structure. For an antigen-presenting cells (APC), there is not any necessity to present antigens to B lymphocytes. Epitopes antigens recognized by T cells are narrow linear peptides from 8 to 20 amino acids [4, 16, 17].

After binding of antigens to the receptors that are membrane- bound antibodies; IgM and IgD type, B lymphocyte become activated. The clonal expansion which means proliferation of antigen specific cells follows the activation of B lymphocytes and they differentiate into antibody-secreting effector cells. The specificity of the naïve B cell membrane-bound antibody receptors is same with the secreted free antibodies. During their differentiation period, some B cells may differentiate to produce antibodies with different heavy chain classes (or isotypes) called as heavy chain class (isotype) switching. After switching, different effector functions can be monitored. Repeated exposure to an antigen leads to the production of antibodies with increasing capacity to bind the antigen; called as affinity maturation [4, 18].

Antibodies responses are classified into two based on the requirement for T cell help; as T-independent or T-dependent

3.1.1. *Antibody responses to T-independent antigens*

If the structure of antigens is non-protein as polysaccharides, lipids, nucleic acids and others antibody responses evoke without the helper T cells participation. These non-protein antigens cannot bind to MHC molecules consequently cannot be detected by T cells.

For immunoglobulin receptor mediated signal transduction in B lymphocytes, the bringing together of two or more antigen molecules in an aggregate (cross-linking), or repeating epitopes of one antigen molecule is needed for antigen binding to membrane bound antibody of the B cell. Multivalent epitope (multiple identical epitopes) as in polysaccharide and lipid antigen can make cross-link many antigen receptors on a specific B cell consequently stimulate proliferation, differentiation and antibody production of B lymphocytes [4, 19].

3.1.2. *Antibody responses to T-dependent antigens*

Most soluble protein antigens cannot make cross-link because they do not contain multivalent epitope so cannot stimulate their proliferation and differentiation of B lymphocytes. Antigen-presenting cells process and helper T lymphocytes remember the protein [5].

Stimulations of two or more protein antigens lead at least three changes in B lymphocytes to improve the interaction of these B cells with helper T lymphocytes.

The changes are:

1. Increased expression of B7 co-stimulator,
2. Increased expression of cytokine receptor
3. Reduced expression of chemokine receptors.

The T cell activation by B cell requires antigen recognition and co-stimulation:

1. Antigen recognition: B lymphocytes work as antigen-presenting cells (APCs); B lymphocytes may bind, internalize and process the antigen protein, and present multiple different peptides of that protein to T lymphocyte.

2. Co-stimulation: The helper T cells are stimulated by B7 molecules as co-stimulator expressed by B cells.

CD40 ligand (CD40) and cytokines are expressed by CD4+ helper T lymphocytes after activation. CD40 ligand; a surface protein delivers the co-stimulatory signal in B cells and interacts with CD40 on the surface of B lymphocytes. Attachment of CD40 and cytokines stimulate B cell clonal expression and antibody production. Class switching and affinity maturation are also stimulated by helper T lymphocytes [4, 5, 19].

After B lymphocytes proliferation and differentiation into antibody-secreting plasma cells, the antibodies enter the blood through lymphoid follicle. Some plasma cells move to bone marrow, live at the bone marrow for months or years and continue to produce antibodies afterwards antigen is removed. These antibodies supply a rapid response when they meet with same antigen. The humoral immune response decreases physiologically by time because of programmed B cell death. But a small number of activated cells differentiate into memory cells, which "freeze" in a state for a very long time [4, 18, 19]. When the body encounter with the same antigen, the memory cells quickly change into antibody-secreting plasma cells and produce immunoglobulins. The two advantages of memory cells;

1. Shorter reaction day: instead of five or more days, it takes one or two.

2. B memory cells differentiate with class switch and somatic hypermutation so in case of reinfection, only memory cells with higher affinities and class switch are selected which are completely same with the B cell receptors of the original infection. Recurring antigen stimulation causes to helper T lymphocytes increase consecutively antibody increase with heavy chain class switching and affinity increase [17, 19].

3.2. Stimuli for generation of autoantibody

Failure of immunologic tolerance can cause the development of autoimmunity. With a genetic background, intolerance can be triggered by environmental factors as sunlight, drugs, chemicals, and infectious agents [5].

1. *Genetic factors*: Immunologic tolerance failure is multifactorial and genetic factors are just one of the cause. For example, the relative risk of having autoimmune disease is 5–50 times higher in siblings of affected individuals than in unrelated ones. Multiple genes; mostly MHC predispose to autoimmune disease and genetic predisposition is detected in many autoimmune diseases. For example, individual with HLA-DR4 gene can be suffered from rheumatoid arthritis but not everyone [5, 6].

2. *Environmental factors*: İnfections can cause the autoimmune diseases by activating self-reactive lymphocytes. The mechanism is like that an infection lead to a local immune response and activation of APCs. Activated APCs secretes co-stimulators - cytokines and

stimulate self-reactive T cells which react with self-antigens in the tissue [4]. Some peptide antigens of microbes are similar to self-antigens, so leads to cross-reactions; called as molecular mimicry [6]. For example; the antibodies against *Porphyromonas gingivalis*; a periodontal pathogen were increased before RA onset and had a relation with RA [20–23].

Microorganisms related autoimmune diseases are listed in **Table 2**.

Sun lights can trigger lupus diseases. Many drugs as procainamide, hydrocarbon pristine, hydralazine, chlorpromazine, methyldopa, quinidine, minocycline and nitrofurantoin can trigger autoimmunity or autoimmune disease through ANAs and ANCAs. Many chemical agents include heavy metals as mercury, gold, and cadmium, pesticides, herbicides, hydrazine can trigger autoimmunity [5].

In organ-specific autoimmune diseases, such as thyroiditis, type 1 diabetes mellitus and primary biliary cirrhosis, autoantibodies can be stimulated by infection of the target organ, through molecular mimicry [16, 24]. In systemic autoimmune diseases, such as systemic lupus, autoantibodies can be triggered by genetic factors. For example; a nuclear autoantibodies produced by antigenic drive from excessive release of death cells antigens and enhanced by intrinsic abnormalities in B or T cells [16, 24].

3.3. Production of autoantibody

3.3.1. Immunologic tolerance

The immune system can differentiate self from non-self [5]. Immunologic tolerance is lack of response to self-antigens that encounter with lymphocytes [6]. The recognition of self is a special set of immune events that all constituents of the organism take a role and may be interrupted by environmental and genetic factors [25–29]. There are three possible immune responses according to antigen type, after antigen encounter with the lymphocytes which has the receptors for a specific antigen;

1. Active immune response: Due to the active lymphocytes and antigen type is called immunogenic. For example, most of non-self-antigens
2. Tolerance: Due to inactive or killed lymphocytes and antigen type is called tolerogenic. For example, self-antigens

Microorganism	Related autoimmune diseases
Streptococcus pyogenes	Rheumatoid fever
Escherichia coli	Primary biliary cirrhosis
Shigella spp.	Reiter syndrome
Hepatitis B	Multiple sclerosis
Coxsackie B4	Type 1 diabetes mellitus
Cytomegalovirus	Scleroderma

Table 2. Infections related with autoimmune diseases.

3. Ignorance: The antigen cannot either stimulate immunity or induce tolerance. This situation is called as ignorance. For example, self-antigens [4, 5].

Immune tolerance is set of immune events, operating both at central immune organs and peripheral ones.

1. Central tolerance happens at immature T and B lymphocytes encounter self-antigens in the thymus and bone marrow.

2. Peripheral tolerance happens at mature lymphocytes encounter self-antigens in peripheral tissues [4, 5].

3.3.2. T lymphocyte tolerance

3.3.2.1. Central T lymphocyte tolerance

The immature T cells die by apoptosis, whenever encounter with self-high avidity protein antigens in the thymus. The immature lymphocytes in the thymus can recognize both self and non-self-antigens. If a self-antigen high in concentration and avidity meet with immature lymphocyte, lymphocytes receives signals that trigger apoptosis, finally dies. This is known as negative selection. Since the self-protein antigens are expressed mainly in thymus because of transcription factor responsible called AIRE (for autoimmune regulator), they are high in concentration [4, 19].

Some lymphocytes which escape from negative selection, mature to dangerous self-reactive T cells with CD4+ T and CD8+ T. They recognize self-antigens through class I and II MHC molecules [4, 18, 19].

And some other develop into regulatory T cells which regulate mostly suppress both naïve and memory T cell responses by a cell to cell contact and by down-regulating the expression of cytokines and co-stimulatory molecules on the antigen-presenting cells. Unfortunately this is not antigen specific reaction [4, 5, 18, 19].

3.3.2.2. Peripheral T lymphocytes tolerance

1. Anergy: Anergy is the functional inactivation of T lymphocytes occurs whenever level of the co-stimulators (second signals) is not enough for T cell activation. If level is enough, the co-stimulatory signal which is taken by CD80 and CD86; interaction of molecules expressed on the surface of APC or B cells, reacts with CD28 (or other receptors) on the T cell surface. If T cells with receptors for the self-antigens encounter with sufficient level of self-antigens (signal 1) but do not receive sufficient signal 2, they may induce long-lived T cell anergy [4, 5, 18, 19].

2. Deletion: Activation-induced cell death: Repeated activation of mature T lymphocytes by repeated encountering with the same antigen cause apoptosis and this is called deletion or activation-induced cell death [4, 18].

3. Immune suppression: Autoreactive mature T lymphocytes that encounter with self-antigen may develop into regulatory cells which suppress the self-reactive lymphocytes response [4, 18, 19].

3.3.2.3. B cell tolerance

If the self-antigens are in structure of polysaccharides, lipids and nucleic acids antigens, they must induce tolerance in B cell and prevent autoantibody production [4]. The B cell tolerance is a set of actions and finally ends with the depletion of or inactive autoreactive B cells. These processes occur at the every stage of B cell [30, 31].

3.4. Central B cell tolerance

When immature B cells encounter with self-antigens in the bone marrow, the B cells are killed and the process is called as negative selection [4].

When immature B cells recognize self-antigens in the bone marrow, they may activate their genes of antibodies and start to express a new light chain. These light chains bind to the previously produced Ig heavy chain to produce a new antigen receptor. This process is called receptor editing. The mechanisms of B cell tolerance are multifaceted and may involve receptor editing, controlled migration, and limited availability of BAFF, CD22, Siglec-G, miRNA, and follicular regulatory T cells [30–33].

3.4.1. Peripheral B cell tolerance

When mature B lymphocytes encounter with high concentration of self-antigens and B cells producing antibodies that bind with high affinity to self-antigens in peripheral lymphoid tissues, they become anergic; functionally inactivation. T cell-independent antigens can trigger strong signals in the B cell. If it is not strong, the B lymphocytes become anergic [30, 34, 35].

3.5. Role of natural autoantibody

Roles of self-reactive B cells are changing according to binding affinities to self-antigens. If self-reactive B cells produce antibodies with high affinity, they undergo elimination or anergy. But if self-reactive B cells produce antibodies with medium or low affinity, they may escape from anergy, even in non-autoimmune individuals [30, 34, 35].Therefore, a significant proportion of immunoglobulins in healthy individuals are made by these autoantibodies. Most of the medium/low affinity antibodies are multireactive and recognize both self and non-self-antigens [30, 35]. They are called as natural antibodies or natural autoantibodies [16, 17, 36]. Because of their multireactivity, the natural antibodies take an important role in the first part of defense against infections [16, 37] and natural autoantibodies in the development of the B cell repertoire [38].

Most of natural autoantibodies are IgM isotype, polyreactive with moderate and low affinity. Therefore, they bind to several unrelated antigens. Also there are natural mono-reactive antibodies [16, 36, 39, 40]. Natural autoantibodies are expressed mostly by CD5+ B1 cell which is the most common B lymphocytes in the neonatal period and in marginal zone B cells [41, 42]. These B1 lymphocytes actively present antigens [43] and also play an important role in the pathogenic autoantibodies production of some autoimmune diseases, as rheumatoid arthritis, Sjögren syndrome, primary antiphospholipid syndrome and systemic lupus [44].

In the infantile periods as an evolutionary process, proteins participate mainly in the building and protection of the organism from non-self and self-antigens. During evolution period, these proteins are highly preserved as the autopolyreactive IgM natural autoantibodies (Nabs) produced mainly by B-1 CD5þ cells [25, 41] and also after class switch, polymeric and monomeric IgG isotype antibodies are produced by mostly B2 cells [25, 45].

Natural antibodies take critical roles; such as:

1. Differentiation self from foreign
2. Recognition of self
3. At evolution period, autopolyreactivity
4. First line defense against non-self-antigens; bacterial and viral infections [46].
5. Regulate the immune system protect the system against tolerance breakdown and the autoimmune diseases.
6. Maintain tissue balance [47]: Up or down regulation of immunotolerance leads to susceptibility/ progressive or protective role in disease as chronic inflammatory disease [48], cancer [49], cardiovascular disease [50], and certain neurodegenerative conditions [33, 34].
7. Clearance of tissue and cell debris after degradation [51]; Most diseases is resulting the destruction of tissues/cells which leads to the continuous antigens release. Natural autoantibody recognizes antigens in cell debris and can react with specific antigens of target tissues. In case of chronic inflammation, more natural autoantibody can be stimulated and some autoantigens can mutate to xenoantigens; after these mutations, more specific pathogenic or protective antibodies can be produced [52].

During cell death, some multiple intracellular enzymes as nucleases and proteases are activated which cause the numerous cellular molecules cleavage; as a consequence, some hidden antigens are exposed and called as 'neoepitopes' or neodeterminants. Most of the neoepitopes are undergo to tolerance, but some undergo modification; as cleavage, phosphorylation and oxidation. The self-antigens released by dying cells can be changed by ultraviolet light, oxidation or cleavage by granzyme B [53] delivered by cytotoxic T cells and this change can lead to autoimmune responses. In rheumatoid arthritis, cyclic citrullinated peptides autoantibodies (anti-CCP antibodies) are one of a neoepitope secondary to inflammation [54]. Citrulline is formed by deamination of the arginine amino acid during inflammation/oxidative stress or apoptosis.

3.6. Generation of pathogenic autoantibody

In specific autoimmune diseases, some of autoantibodies could be detected before beginning of the disease. For example; in SLE, rheumatoid arthritis, type I diabetes, limbic encephalitis and primary biliary cholangitis [55].

Changing from preclinical to clinical autoantibody has certain steps. In genetic predisposed individuals, autoantibodies are produced by autoreactive cells. These preclinical autoantibodies can stay for months or even years in these individuals. Under proper environmental conditions, the autoreactive cells would be activated and proliferated. Then, they produce large amounts of autoantibodies and inflammatory cytokines, which lead to tissue injury and the clinical symptoms are observed [6].

Natural autoantibodies can provide the templates for the higher-affinity and class-switched pathogenic autoantibodies, under appropriate conditions [16].

Production of pathogenic autoantibody:

1. Somatic hypermutation: Each antibody can bind at least 2 (IgG, IgD and IgE isotypes) – maximum 10 epitopes (IgM isotype) of an antigen, which has identical epitopes and are close enough. If the multiple antigen-antibody bind each other, the total strength of the bond is much greater than a single one. This is called the avidity of the interaction. The molar concentration of an antigen needed to occupy half the available antibody molecules in a solution is the dissociation constant (Kd) and used for expression of affinity. The lower the Kd means the higher the affinity. In a primary immune response, produced antibodies have a Kd in the range of 10^{-6}–10^{-9} M and after encountering with repeated antigens, the affinity can rises up to 10–11 M. This increase in antigen-binding strength is called affinity maturation or somatic hypermutation [4]. Mostly point mutations in the genes responsible for variable regions of antibody are detected [16]. They happen in the germinal centers of secondary follicles and AID enzyme that initiate them [17].

2. Class switching: The membrane bound IgM and IgD the antigen receptors of naïve B lymphocytes. After stimulation, the antigen specific clone B lymphocytes may proliferate and differentiate into antibody-secreting cells. Some of these B cells may secrete IgM, and some others may produce antibodies of other heavy chain classes. The change in Ig isotype production is called heavy chain class switching. The V regions remains same, specificity of B cells maintains [4].

The exons encoding the constant regions of all antibody classes on chromosome 14, are placed with μ (for IgM) nearest to variable region segments, followed by γ (IgG), α (IgA) and ε (IgE). By a successful VDJ rearrangement, first the nearest constant region which is μ is used, resulting in the production of IgM [17]. Unmutated or minimally mutated recombined VDJ gene sequences encode the multi and monoreactive natural IgM antibodies/autoantibodies [56]. AID deaminates cytidines in immunoglobulin VDJ and switch-region DNA, then ssDNA nicks, gaps or double-strand breaks are generated. Repair of these lesions involving error-prone translesion DNA polymerases are made by the B cell DNA and this results in insertions of point mutations or resolution of double-strand breaks, and hence, class-switch DNA recombination [57]. After class switch with the same variable region, these cells can express IgG if the exons encoding the γ constant region; IgA if it is α constant region; and IgE if it is ε constant region. T-lymphocytes and other cells release cytokines influence isotype of class switch [17].

Unmutated natural IgM autoantibodies expressed by B1 cells provide the 'templates' for the high-affinity and class-switched IgG and/or IgA autoantibodies which can cause autoimmune diseases [49, 58, 59]. Anti-DNA, anti-insulin and anti-IgG (RF) autoantibodies are pathogenic high-affinity autoantibodies that undergo somatic hypermutation, class-switch DNA recombination and antigen driven clonal selection detected at systemic lupus, type 1 diabetes and rheumatoid arthritis patients [60]. Somatic hypermutation and class-switching [56, 60, 61] including the expression of activation-induced cytidine deaminase (AID) [62] are associated with the expansion of B-2 cells.

Class switch and somatic hypermutation are initiated by the same enzyme, AID, in the germinal centers of secondary follicles parallelly [17].

3. Somatic diversity: Somatic recombination: Antibodies are capable of binding a wide variety of antigen, since variable region of antibody molecules forms a flat surface field into different shapes. The epitopes or determinants are the parts of antigens that are recognized by antibodies based on sequence (linear determinants) or shape (conformational determinants). Some hidden antigen molecules are exposed after a physicochemical change, called as neodeterminants [4].

Diversity of antibodies is generated by the genetics arrangement of antibody production; unique molecular random generator. The variable region of an immunoglobulin is formed by both the heavy and the light chain which are carried on different chromosomes [5]. The variable portion of the heavy chain is encoded in separated gene segments of three types, V (variable; the number of gene segments is 65), D (diversity; 27) and J (joining; 6). A complete heavy chain variable region exon is randomly cobbled together by juxtaposing one V, one D and one J segment by a cut and paste process at the DNA level by an enzyme complex containing RAG-proteins (recombination activating gene) which excises intervening DNA, and normal DNA repair proteins directly rejoin the segments. Light chain genes have just V and J segments, not D [17]. In summary, the diversity of antigen binding is achieved by mostly V genes and their combination with different D and J genes. Different antibodies are produced by four different mechanisms as; randomly combining V-(D)-J segments, randomly combining heavy and light chain, imprecise joining and somatic hypermutation [4, 17]. Somatic diversity is performed during central B cell intolerance.

4. Genetic abnormalities: Some genetic alterations results clinical autoimmune disease but some alterations are influenced by environmental factors. For example; single gen knockout and overexpression lead to clinical autoimmune disease while most of the autoimmune disorders are polygenic. Three examples of spontaneous or induced genetic alterations lead to clinical diseases [16].

a. Abnormal survival of autoreactive lymphocytes: Mutations in Fas/CD95 causes over expression of the B cell stimulator BLyS; BAFF and the antiapoptotic regulator Bcl-2 which leads the abnormal survival of autoreactive lymphocytes. It causes an autoimmune lymphoproliferative syndrome/Canale Smith syndrome in humans [16, 63],

b. Defective removal of apoptotic cells: A group of proteins as Mer and serum opsonins (e.g., natural IgM antibodies, C1q, serum amyloid P component [SAP] and milk fat globulin epithelial growth factor-8 [MFGE8]) [64] take role in the removal of apoptotic cells. In Mer deficiency, macrophages take a proinflammatory signal not an anti-inflammatory one for ingestion of apoptotic cells. If there is a defective clearance of apoptotic cells in surface IgM, C1q, SAP and MFGE8, clearance of apoptotic cells leads to postapoptotic necrosis and/or through lack of engagement with specific inhibitory receptors on the phagocyte. In

MFG-E8 deficiency, apoptotic cells accumulate in germinal centers and in C1q-deficiency, apoptotic cells accumulate in the kidney. These deficiencies cause lupus-like diseases [16].

c. Breakdown in the regulation of B cell or T cell activation threshold: If threshold regulators of cbl-b, PD-1 and Zap-70 and the SLAM cluster in T cells, and Lyn and FcγRIIb in B cells change genetically, failure of peripheral immune system could happens. If lymphocytes are more easily activated, they produce more auto-antibodies as in systemic lupus. Mutations of Zap-70 lead to production of RFs as in rheumatoid arthritis [16, 65]. PD-1-deficiency causes lupus in C57BL/6 and myocarditis in BALB/c.

There is some signature autoantibodies cause autoimmune diseases as anti-endomysial antibodies (EMA), anti-gliadin antibodies (AGA). But there is not a specific antibody detected yet in several autoimmune diseases, as psoriasis [6].

Lymphocytes and APC are strongly activated by type I interferons (interferon-α and β) [66]. Patients with systemic lupus have elevated levels of interferon and autoantibodies as anti-DNA and Sm/RNP. By binding to chromatin which contains DNA or to Sm/RNP which contain small nuclear RNAs, they enter cells through the FcγR or B cell receptor. The intracellular Toll-like receptor is activated by nucleic acid which leads to production of interferon and activation of immune system. The protein antigen stimulates T cells, probably are responsible for the specificity of the immune response. These are called Toll hypothesis [67].

3.7. Systemic versus organ-specific autoimmune disease

Autoimmune disease can be classified as systemic or organ specific. Systemic autoimmune diseases (**Table 3**), involve multiple organs or tissues, whereas organ specific autoimmune

Disease	Organ(s) involved	Autoantibodies
Systemic lupus erythematosus	Joints, skin, nervous system, kidneys, blood cells, heart, lungs	Anti dsDNAb Anti Sm b Anti ribosomal P b Anti RNA helicase
Rheumatoid arthritis	Joints, blood, vessels, lungs	Anti citrullinated peptides b Rheumatoid factor
Sjögren's syndrome	Exocrine glands (salivary and lacrimal glands), kidneys, nerves	Anti Ro60 (SS-A) Anti Ro52 Anti La (SS-B)
Scleroderma	Skin, blood vessels, GI tract, lungs, kidneys	Anti topoisomerase I b Anti fi brillarin (U3 RNP) b Anti RNA polymerase I b Anti RNA polymerase III b
Polymyositis	Muscles, lungs	tRNA synthetases (Histidyl, alanyl, threonyl, glycyl, etc.) b Signal recognition particle b

Table 3. Some systemic autoimmune diseases.

Disease	Organ(s) involved	Autoantibodies
Hashimoto's thyroiditis	Thyroid	Thyroid peroxidase Thyroglobulin
Graves' disease	Thyroid	Thyroid-stimulating hormone receptor
Addison's disease	Adrenal glands	2I-hydroxylase
Type I diabetes	Pancreatic islet cells	Glutamic acid dehydrogenase, insulin islet cell antigens
Pemphigus vulgaris	Skin	Desmoglein 3
Bullous pemphigoid	Skin	230 kDa hemidesmosomal antigen
Vitiligo	Skin melanocytes	Unknown melanocyte antigens
Goodpasture's syndrome	Kidneys, lungs	Type VII collagen
Myasthenia gravis	Nervous system	Acetylcholine receptor
Multiple sclerosis	Nervous system	Unknown myelin antigens
Pernicious anemia	Gastric parietal cells	Parietal cell antigens, intrinsic factor
Primary biliary cirrhosis	Bile ducts	Dihydrolipoamide acyltransferase and other antigens b
Autoimmune hepatitis	Liver	Smooth muscle antigens (F-actin)

Table 4. Some organ-specific autoimmune diseases.

diseases (**Table 4**), involve a single organ or tissue. Almost all organs can be affected by either systemic or organ-specific autoimmune disease [5].

4. Function of autoantibodies; mechanism of protection and cause of diseases?

The antibodies' Fab regions bind to antigens and can block/stimulate the effects of them and the Fc regions can bind to many cells of immune system as phagocytes and complement and activate diverse effector mechanisms to eliminate these antigens; Fcγ-R (for IgG), Fcα-R (for IgA), Fcα/μ-R (for IgA and IgM), Fcε-R (for IgE). The effective binding of antigen-antibody occurs after recognization several IgG molecules. The affinity of the binding is too low with a single, free antibody. Bigger immune complexes by antigen and several Fc parts of antibodies causes to rapid internalization for phagocytosis and antigen clearance. Heavy chain class switching and affinity maturation enhance the protective functions of antibodies. There is an exception to this rule in mast cells and eosinophils, just binding a free (meaning non-antigen-complexed) IgE is enough because of their high-affinity Fc-ε-receptors [4, 17].

4.1. Some examples for the functions of antibodies and autoantibodies

1. Neutralization of foreign and self-antigens: Antibodies bind to block, or neutralize the activity of foreign or self-antigens [4].

2. Opsonization and phagocytosis: Complex of antibodies with foreign and self-antigens promote their ingestion by phagocytes (opsonization). When IgG1 and IgG3 isotype antibodies bind to a foreign or self-antigen, their Fc regions bind to a high affinity receptors called FcγRI (CD64), which are on neutrophils and macrophages. The binding of antibody Fc tails to FcγRI results in opsonization of antigenic molecules into a vesicle called a phagosome, where fuse with lysosomes and activates the neutrophil or phagocytes. The activated ones produces in their lysosomes, large amounts of reactive oxygen intermediates, nitric oxide, and proteolytic enzymes, all of them together destroy the ingested antigenic cells [4].

3. Antibody-dependent cellular cytotoxicity (ADCC): Natural killer (NK) cells produce an Fc receptor called FcγRIII, which binds to IgG antibodies. The activated NK cells discharge their granules, which contains proteins that kill the opsonized targets [4]

4. Activation of the complement system: Antigens without antibody, as part of innate immune response to infection, and antigens with antibody, as part of adaptive immunity can activate the complement system. The complement system takes role in the elimination of opsonized antigens [4]. Examples; activation of complement causes diseases at kidneys of systemic lupus and lupus nephritis patients, fetal loss associated with the antiphospholipid syndrome [68, 69], autoantibody administration into the transgenic K/BxN mouse of rheumatoid arthritis [70], in glucose-6-phosphate isomerase patient. In the NZB/W F1 murine model of immune-complex-mediated lupus nephritis, mice lacking the FcγRγ chain were protected from nephritis, indicating a critical role for FcγRs in tissue inflammation [71].

5. Mucosal immunity.

6. Pro-inflammatory and anti-inflammatory effect: natural polyautoreactive IgM antibodies can protect from autoimmune diseases [30]. Also IgG isotype autoantibodies has an anti-inflammatory capacities, according to their IgG subclass and the extent of glycosylation/sialylation of the Fc glycan linked to Asn297 [71, 72]. These properties regulate the binding of antibody to a different Fc-receptors [72]. The receptors as FcγRI (CD64), FcγRIIIA (CD16a), and FcγRIIIB (CD16b) mediate activating signals, but also FcγRIIA and FcγRIIB (CD32) mediate inhibiting signals. Glycosylated/ sialylated different IgG isotypes antibodies bind to Fc-receptors for activating and inhibiting with different affinities [72]. According to glycosylation/sialylation patterns and IgG subclass determine, an autoantibody produces FcγR-mediated either pro- or anti-inflammatory functions [73]. So glycosylation of autoantibody can be an important regulator of autoimmune disorders [74]. While IgG isotypes produced with T cell-dependent reactions were poorly sialylated causes pro- inflammatory, a high degree of sialylation that mediates anti-inflammatory properties [75]. Activated B cells and plasma cells regulate both T cell differentiation into follicular helper T cells and cytokine profiles [76]. By stimulation of TLR, B lymphocytes produce different cytokines to dendritic cells [77]. Dendritic cells are the most important antigen-presenting cells to T cell. B cell also present the antigen to T cell and so promote the proliferation of activated T lymphocytes, the development of robust T effector responses, and normal T cell memory compartments [78]. TLR-signals in murine B cells promote IFN-γ production from T cells and control antibody isotype switching to IgG2 *in vivo* [77]. The cowork of activated B and T cells is crucial for the antibody responses and their outcome as pathogenic potential, that is, the antibody class and glycosylation/sialylation pattern.

Testing of autoantibodies is diagnostic criteria in many diseases. But, also autoantibodies could be detected in healthy individuals [79]. Since isotype/subclass and glycosylation pattern is critical for the pathogenic potential of a particular antibody, it could be helpful for the diagnostic analysis. Pathogenic autoantibodies could be produced either by continuous formation of short-lived plasma cells or through the formation of long-lived plasma cells, or both [80]. Therapeutic treatment available nowadays could suppress B cell activation and short-lived plasma cell, while do nothing to long-lived plasma cells [81].

By contrast, mice with FcγRIIb knocked out spontaneously develop a lupus like disease [71]. Different isotypes antibodies have different affinities for the four FcγRs. IgG2a has higher affinity for FcγRIV, leading to inflammatory responses, whereas IgG1 selectively engages FcγRIIb, leading to inhibitory responses [30]. There is a similar relationships with human FcγRs and that the ability to protect or induce inflammation will change according to the isotype of the autoantibody and FcγR engaged.

7. Removal of cell debris: Natural autoantibodies takes role in the removal of cell debris during inflammation, and autoantibodies to inflammatory cytokines have protective functions against inflammation [82].

4.2. Mechanisms of autoimmune tissue injury

Immune responses can cause tissue injury and disorders called as hypersensitivity diseases. Hypersensitivity is a term of excessive or aberrant immune responses [4]. Tissue damage in autoimmune diseases can occur through several mechanisms, which are similar to three of the classical types of hypersensitivity reactions [5]:

1. Type II (caused by autoantibodies reactive with cell surface or matrix antigens):

Antibodies against cell and tissue may cause tissue and disease. IgM and IgG antibodies activate the phagocytosis of cells by binding to complement and Fc receptor- mediated leukocyte [4]. The reactions are caused by antibodies against self-protein antigens. Autoantibodies generated against cell surface antigens/extracellular matrix proteins may be cytotoxic (type IIA) or agonistic/antagonistic (type IIB). Autoantibodies to cell surface antigens may initiate cell destruction by complement- mediated lysis (cell destruction), phagocytosis, or antibody-dependent cell-mediated cytotoxicity (ADCC) [5]. At **Table 5**, some examples of antibody-mediated diseases are given.

Disease	Target antigen	Mechanism
Pemphigus vulgaris	Proteins in intercellular junction of epidermal cell	Antibody-mediated activation of proteinase, disruption of intercellular adhesion
Autoimmune hemolytic anemia	Erythrocytes membrane antigen	Opsonization and phagocytosis of erythrocytes
Myasthenia gravis	Acetylcholine receptor	Antibody inhibits acetylcholine binding

Table 5. Antibody-mediated diseases.

2. Type III (caused by immune complexes):

Autoantibodies can bind to circulating antigens and form immune complexes that deposit in vessels, tissues and cause tissue injury. Injury is mainly due to leukocyte recruitment and inflammation [4]. Autoantibodies can cause disease by forming immune complexes with the circulating antigens. Immune complex formation is a normal process to remove antigens and to phagocyte through Fc or complement receptors so are prevented their deposition. The efficiency of uptake of immune complexes by either Fc receptors or CR1 is proportional to the number of IgG molecules associated in the complex [5]. At **Table 6**, some examples of immune complex mediated diseases are given.

3. Type IV (delayed-type hypersensitivity, mediated by T cells):

T cell-mediated disease is caused by CD4 T lymphocytes or by killing of host cells by CD8 CTLs [4]. T cells recognize protein antigen-presenting cells in the context of class II major histocompatibility complex (MHC) molecules and produce the cytokines interferon γ (IFN-γ), interleukin 3 (IL-3), tumor necrosis factor (TNF) α, TNF-β, and granulocyte-macrophage colony-stimulating factor (GM-CSF). Elaboration of "TH1 (a subset of helper T cells) cytokines" leads to macrophage recruitment and activation, enhanced expression of adhesion molecules, and increased production of monocytes by the bone marrow [5]. At **Table 7**, some examples of T cell-mediated diseases are given.

Disease	Target antigen	Mechanism
Systemic lupus erythematosus	DNA, nucleoproteins	Complement and Fc region mediated
Polyarteritis nodosa	Hepatitis B surface antigen	Complement and Fc region mediated
Poststreptococcal glomerulonephritis	Streptococcal cell wall antigen	Complement and Fc region mediated

Table 6. Immune complex mediated diseases.

Disease	Target antigen	Mechanism
Rheumatoid arthritis	Antigen in joint synovium	T cell mediated
Type I diabetes mellitus	Islet cell antigen	T cell mediated

Table 7. T cell-mediated diseases.

Author details

Neval Yurttutan Uyar

Address all correspondence to: nevaluyar@gmail.com

Mehmet Ali Aydınlar Acibadem University, Istanbul, Turkey

References

[1] Bach JF. The effect of infections on susceptibility to autoimmune and allergic diseases. The New England Journal of Medicine. 2002;**347**:911-920. DOI: 10.1056/NEJMra020100

[2] Vento S, Cainelli F. Autommune diseases in low and middle income countries: A neglected issue in global health. The Israel Medical Association Journal. 2016;**18**(1):54-55

[3] Eaton WW, Rose NR, Kalaydjian A, Pedersen MG, Mortensen PB. Epidemiology of autoimmune diseases in Denmark. Journal of Autoimmunity. 2007;**29**:1-9. DOI: 10.1016/j.jaut.2007.05.002

[4] Abbas AK, Lichtman AH. Basic Immunology–Functions and Disorders of Immune System. 2nd ed. Saunder; 2004. p 300. ISBN:0-7216-0241-X

[5] Zabriskie J.B. Essential Clinical Immunology. 2nd ed. Cambridge; 2009. p 362. ISBN-13 978-0-521-51681-5

[6] Ma W, Chang C, Gershwin ME, Lian Z. Development of autoantibodies precedes clinical manifestations ofautoimmune diseases: A comprehensive review. Journal of Autoimmunity. 2017;**83**:95-112. DOI: 10.1016/j.jaut.2017.07.003

[7] Cruz GI et al. A Child's HLA-DRB1 genotype increases maternal risk ofsystemic lupus erythematosus. Journal of Autoimmunity. 2016;**74**:201-207

[8] Ji J, Sundquist J, Sundquist K. Gender-specific incidence of autoimmune diseases from national registers. Journal of Autoimmunity. 2016;**69**:102-106

[9] Long H et al. The critical role of epigenetics in systemic lupus erythematosus and autoimmunity. Journal of Autoimmunity. 2016;**74**:118-138

[10] Teruel M, Alarcon-Riquelme ME. The genetic basis of systemic lupus erythematosus: What are the risk factors and what have we learned. Journal of Autoimmunity. 2016;**74**: 161-175

[11] Bao Y, Cao X. Epigenetic control of B cell development and B-cell-related immune disorders. Clinical Reviews in Allergy and Immunology. 2016;**50**(3):301-311

[12] Floreani A, Leung PS, Gershwin ME. Environmental basis of autoimmunity. Clinical Reviews in Allergy & Immunology. 2016;**50**(3):287-300

[13] Meroni PL, Penatti AE. Epigenetics and systemic lupus erythematosus: Unmet needs. Clinical Reviews in Allergy and Immunology. 2016;**50**(3):367-376

[14] Selmi C. Autoimmunity in 2015. Clinical Reviews in Allergy and Immunology. 2016;**51**(1): 110-119

[15] Wu HJ et al. Critical link between epigenetics and transcription factors in the induction of autoimmunity: A comprehensive review. Clinical Reviews in Allergy and Immunology. 2016;**50**(3):333-344

[16] Elkon K, Casali P. Nature and functions of autoantibodies. Nature Clinical Practice. Rheumatology. 2008 September;**4**(9):491-498. DOI: 10.1038/ncprheum0895

[17] Helmberg A. Immune system and immunology [Internet]. 2014. Available from: http://www.helmberg.at/immunology.htm

[18] Us A.D. Temel İmmunoloji ve Seroloji. 1st ed. Hipokrat Kitabevi. P367. ISBN:978-605-9160-39-1

[19] Levinson W. Review of Medical Microbiology and Immunology. 14th ed. Lange; 2013. p818. ISBN:978-0-07-184574-8

[20] Uhlig T, Hagen KB, Kvien TK. Current tobacco smoking, formal education, and the risk of rheumatoid arthritis. The Journal of Rheumatology. 1999;**26**(1):47-54

[21] Heliovaara M et al. Smoking and risk of rheumatoid arthritis. The Journal of Rheumatology. 1993;**20**(11):1830-1835

[22] Kharlamova N et al. Antibodies to *Porphyromonas gingivalis* indicate interaction between oral infection, smoking, and risk genes in rheumatoid arthritis etiology. Arthritis & Rhematology. 2016;**68**(3):604-613

[23] Johansson L et al. Concentration of antibodies against *Porphyromonas gingivalis* is increased before the onset of symptoms of rheumatoid arthritis. Arthritis Research & Therapy. 2016:18

[24] Kaklıkkaya N, Kaşifoğlu N, Sarıbaş Z, Şener B, Taşkınoğlu T, Yurttutan Uyar N. Klinik Örnekten Sonuç Raporuna Uygulama Rehberi. 2nd ed. Çağlayan offset; 2016. p152. ISBN: 978-605-84108-4-8

[25] Avrameas S, Selmi C. Natural autoantibodies in the physiology and pathophysiology of the immune system. Journal of Autoimmunity. 2013;**41**:46-49. DOI: 10.1016/j.jaut.2013.01.006

[26] Miller FW, Alfredsson L, Costenbader KH, Kamen DL, Nelson LM, Norris JM, et al. Epidemiology of environmental exposures and human autoimmune diseases: Findings from a National Institute of Environmental Health Sciences Expert Panel Workshop. Journal of Autoimmunity. 2012;**39**:259-271

[27] Selmi C, Leung PS, Sherr DH, Diaz M, Nyland JF, Monestier M, et al. Mechanisms of environmental influence on human autoimmunity: A National Institute Of Environmental Health Sciences Expert Panel Workshop. Journal of Autoimmunity. 2012;**39**:272-284

[28] Miller FW, Pollard KM, Parks CG, Germolec DR, Leung PS, Selmi C, et al. Criteria for environmentally associated autoimmune diseases. Journal of Autoimmunity. 2012;**39**:253-258

[29] Germolec D, Kono DH, Pfau JC, Pollard KM. Animal models used to examine the role of the environment in the development of autoimmune disease: Findings from an NIEHS expert panel workshop. Journal of Autoimmunity. 2012;**39**:285-293

[30] Ralf J, Ludwig RJ, Vanhoorelbeke K, Leypoldt F, Kaya Z, Bieber K, McLachlan SM, Komorowski L, Luo J, Cabral-Marques O, Hammers CM, Lindstrom JM, Lamprecht P, Fischer A, Riemekasten G, Tersteeg C, Sondermann P, Rapoport B, Wandinger KP, Probst C, Beidaq AE, Schmidt E, Verkman A, Manz RA, Nimmerjahn F. Mechanisms of autoantibody-induced pathology. Frontiers in Immunology. **8**:603. DOI: 10.3389/fimmu.2017.00603

[31] Pelanda R, Torres RM. Central B-cell tolerance: Where selection begins. Cold Spring Harbor Perspectives in Biology. 2012;**4**:a007146. DOI: 10.1101/cshperspect.a007146

[32] Gonzalez-Martin A, Adams BD, Lai M, Shepherd J, Salvador-Bernaldez M, Salvador JM, et al. The microRNA miR-148a functions as a critical regulator of B cell tolerance and autoimmunity. Nature Immunology. 2016;**17**:433-440. DOI: 10.1038/ni.3385

[33] Müller J, Nitschke L. The role of CD22 and Siglec-G in B-cell tolerance and autoimmune disease. Nature Reviews Rheumatology. 2014;**10**:422-428. DOI: 10.1038/ nrrheum.2014.54

[34] Tiller T, Tsuiji M, Yurasov S, Velinzon K, Nussenzweig MC, Wardemann H. Autoreactivity in human IgG+ memory B cells. Immunity. 2007;**26**:205-213. DOI: 10.1016/j.immuni.2007.01.009

[35] Wardemann H, Yurasov S, Schaefer A, Young JW, Meffre E, Nussenzweig MC. Predominant autoantibody production by early human B cell precursors. Science. 2003;**301**:1374-1377. DOI: 10.1126/science.1086907

[36] Avrameas S. Natural autoantibodies: From 'horror autotoxicus' to 'gnothi seauton'. Immunology Today. 1991;**12**:154-159

[37] Carroll MC. The lupus paradox. Nature Genetics. 1998;**19**:3-59. [PubMed: 9590274]

[38] Yurasov S, Nussenzweig MC. Regulation of autoreactive antibodies. Current Opinion in Rheumatology. 2007;**19**:421-426. [PubMed: 17762605]

[39] Spalter SH, Kaveri SV, Bonnin E, Mani JC, Cartron JP, Kazatchkine MD. Normal human serum contains natural antibodies reactive with autologous ABO blood group antigens. Blood. 1999;**93**:4418e24

[40] Ravindranath MH, Kaneku H, El-Awar N, Morales-Buenrostro LE, Terasaki PI. Antibodies to HLA-E in nonalloimmunized males: Pattern of HLA-Ia reactivity of anti-HLA--E-positive sera. Journal of Immunology. 2010;**185**:1935e48

[41] Baumgarth N. The double life of a B-1 cell: Self-reactivity selects for protective effector functions. Nature Reviews. Immunology. 2011;**11**:34e46

[42] Tiller T, Tsuiji M, Yurasov S, Velinzon K, Nussenzweig MC, Wardemann H. Autoreactivity in human IgGþ memory B cells. Immunity. 2007;**26**:205e13

[43] Tumas-Brundage KM, Notidis E, Heltemes L, Zhang X, Wysocki LJ, Manser T. Predominance of a novel splenic B cell population in mice expressing a transgene that encodes multireactive antibodies: Support for additional heterogeneity of the B cell compartment. International Immunology. 2001;**13**:475e84

[44] Roy B, Shukla S, Lyszkiewicz M, Krey M, Viegas N, Duber S, et al. Somatic hypermutation in peritoneal B1b cells. Molecular Immunology. 2009;**46**:1613e9

[45] Notkins AL. Polyreactivity of antibody molecules. Trends in Immunology. 2004;**25**:174-179

[46] Zhou ZH et al. The broad antibacterial activity of the natural antibody repertoire is due to polyreactive antibodies. Cell Host & Microbe. 2007;**1**:51-61

[47] Shoenfeld Y, Toubi E. Protective autoantibodies: Role in homeostasis, clinical importance, and therapeutic potential. Arthritis and Rheumatism. 2005;**52**:2599-2606

[48] Chen Y, Khanna S, Goodyear CS, Park YB, Raz E, Thiel S, et al. Regulation of dendritic cells and macrophages by an anti-apoptotic cell natural antibody that suppresses TLR responses and inhibits inflammatory arthritis. Journal of Immunology. 2009;**183**:1346-1359

[49] Toubi E, Shoenfeld Y. Protective autoimmunity in cancer (review). Oncology Reports. 2007;**17**:245-251

[50] de Faire U, Frostegard J. Natural antibodies against phosphorylcholine in cardiovascular disease. Annals of the New York Academy of Sciences. 2009;**1173**:292-300

[51] Grabar P. Some considerations of the problem of auto-antibody formation. Texas Reports on Biology and Medicine. 1965;**23**(Suppl. 1):278-284

[52] Zelenay S et al. Physiopathology of natural auto-antibodies: The case for regulation. Journal of Autoimmunity. 2007;**29**:229-235

[53] Casciola-Rosen L et al. Cleavage by granzyme B is strongly predictive of autoantigen status: Implications for initiation of autoimmunity. The Journal of Experimental Medicine. 1999;**190**:815-826. [PubMed: 10499920]

[54] Klareskog L et al. Genes, environment and immunity in the development of rheumatoid arthritis. Current Opinion in Immunology. 2006;**18**:867-875

[55] Arbuckle MR et al. Development of autoantibodies before the clinical onset of systemic lupus erythematosus. The New England Journal of Medicine. 2003;**349**(16):1526-1533

[56] Harindranath N et al. Structure of the VH and VL segments of polyreactive and monoreactive human natural antibodies to HIV-1 and *Escherichia coli* β-galactosidase. International Immunology. 1993;**5**:1523-1533. [PubMed: 8312222]

[57] Diaz M, Casali P. Somatic immunoglobulin hypermutation. Current Opinion in Immunology. 2002;**14**:235-240. [PubMed: 11869898]

[58] Carroll MC, Prodeus AP. Linkages of innate and adaptive immunity. Current Opinion in Immunology. 1998;**10**:36-40. [PubMed: 9523108]

[59] Zhang M, Carroll MC. Natural antibody mediated innate autoimmune response. Molecular Immunology. 2007;**44**:103-110. [PubMed: 16876247]

[60] Mantovani L et al. Human rheumatoid B-1a (CD5+ B) cells make somatically hypermutated high affinity IgM rheumatoid factors. Journal of Immunology. 1993;**151**: 473-488. [PubMed: 7686945]

[61] Casali P, Schettino EW. Structure and function of natural antibodies. Current Topics in Microbiology and Immunology. 1996;**210**:167-179. [PubMed: 8565555]

[62] Honjo T et al. AID: How does it aid antibody diversity? Immunity 2004;**20**:659-668. [PubMed: 15189732]

[63] Straus SE et al. An inherited disorder of lymphocyte apoptosis: The autoimmune lymphoproliferative syndrome. Annals of Internal Medicine. 1999;**130**:591-601. [PubMed: 10189330]

[64] Peng Y et al. The role of IgM antibodies in the recognition and clearance of apoptotic cells. Molecular Immunology. 2005;**42**:781-787. [PubMed: 15829266]

[65] Sakaguchi N, et al. Altered thymic T-cell selection due to a mutation of the ZAP-70 gene causes autoimmune arthritis in mice. Nature. 2003;**426**:454-460. [PubMed: 14647385]

[66] Theofilopoulos AN, et al. Type I interferons (alpha/beta) in immunity and autoimmunity. Annual Review of Immunology. 2005;**23**:307-336. [PubMed: 15771573]

[67] Martin DA, Elkon KB. Autoantibodies make a U-turn: The toll hypothesis for autoantibody specificity. The Journal of Experimental Medicine. 2005;**202**:1465-1469. [PubMed: 16330812]

[68] Monach PA et al. The role of antibodies in mouse models of rheumatoid arthritis, and relevance to human disease. Advances in Immunology. 2004;**82**:217-248. [PubMed: 14975258]

[69] Baxendale HE, et al. Natural human antibodies to pneumococcus have distinctive molecular characteristics and protect against pneumococcal disease. Clinical and Experimental Immunology. 2008;**151**:51-60. [PubMed: 17983446]

[70] Clynes R, et al. Uncoupling of immune complex formation and kidney damage in autoimmune glomerulonephritis. Science. 1998;**279**:1052-1054. [PubMed: 9461440]

[71] Bolland S, Ravetch JV. Spontaneous autoimmune disease in Fc(gamma)RIIB-deficient mice results from strain-specific epistasis. Immunity. 2000;**13**:277-285. [PubMed: 10981970]

[72] Nimmerjahn F, Ravetch JV. Anti-inflammatory actions of intravenous immunoglobulin. Annual Review of Immunology. 2008;**26**:513-533. DOI: 10.1146/annurev. immunol.26. 021607.090232

[73] Anthony RM, Ravetch JV. A novel role for the IgG Fc glycan: The anti- inflammatory activity of sialylated IgG Fcs. Journal of Clinical Immunology. 2010;**30**(Suppl 1):S9-S14. DOI: 10.1007/s10875-010-9405-6

[74] Goulabchand R et al. Impact of autoantibody glycosylation in autoimmune diseases. Autoimmunity Reviews. 2014;**13**:742-750. DOI: 10.1016/j.autrev.2014.02.005

[75] Hess C et al. T cell-independent B cell activation induces immunosuppressive sialylated IgG antibodies. The Journal of Clinical Investigation. 2013;**123**:3788-3796. DOI:10.1172/JCI65938

[76] Fillatreau S, Gray D, Anderton SM. Not always the bad guys: B cells as regulators of autoimmune pathology. Nature Reviews. Immunology. 2008;**8**:391-397. DOI: 10.1038/nri2315

[77] Barr TA, Brown S, Ryan G, Zhao J, Gray D. TLR-mediated stimulation of APC: Distinct cytokine responses of B cells and dendritic cells. European Journal of Immunology. 2007;**37**:3040-3053. DOI: 10.1002/eji.200636483

[78] Crawford A et al. Primary T cell expansion and differentiation in vivo requires antigen presentation by B cells. Journal of Immunology. 2006;**176**:3498-3506. DOI: 10.4049/jimmunol.176.6.3498

[79] Nagele EP et al. Natural IgG autoantibodies are abundant and ubiquitous in human sera, and their number is influenced by age, gender, and disease. PLoS One. 2013;**8**:e60726. DOI: 10.1371/journal.pone.0060726

[80] Manz RA, Hauser AE, Hiepe F, Radbruch A. Maintenance of serum anti-body levels. Annual Review of Immunology. 2005;**23**:367-386. DOI: 10.1146/annurev. immunol.23.021704.115723

[81] Mumtaz IM, et al. Bone marrow of NZB/W mice is the major site for plasma cells resistant to dexamethasone and cyclophosphamide: Implications for the treatment of autoimmunity. Journal of Autoimmunology. 2012;**39**:180-188. Doi:10.1016/j.jaut.2012.05.010

[82] Wildbaum G, et al. Beneficial autoimmunity to proinflammatory mediators restrains the consequences of self-destructive immunity. Immunity. 2003;**19**:679-688. [PubMed: 14614855]

Chapter 3

Autoantibodies: Key Mediators of Autoimmune Infertility

Kaushiki M. Kadam, Purvi Mande and
Asmita Choudhury

Additional information is available at the end of the chapter

http://dx.doi.org/10.5772/intechopen.73899

Abstract

Autoimmune diseases have gender bias with predominance in females, autoimmune infertility (AI) being no exception. This chapter will focus on AI in females with brief reference to the same in males. Autoimmune diseases have established protocols for detection and management of ensuing infertility, however similar protocols for unexplained infertility [tubal blockage, endometriosis, premature ovarian insufficiency (POI), undiagnosed underlying autoimmune disease (Sjögren's syndrome, IBS, celiac disease) and tubal blockage] are not established. Endometriosis and POI, in particular, have autoimmune etiology yet lack specific and sensitive biomarkers for accurate diagnosis. If autoantibodies are indeed diagnosed, then treatment regimen focuses on AI which has known adverse effects. The detection of natural antibodies as autoantibodies presents a viable alternative to organ specific biomarker panel for better management of AI.

Keywords: autoantibodies, premature ovarian insufficiency, endometriosis, autoimmune infertility

1. Introduction

As per *immunculus* concept, natural antibodies (NAbs) are formed in response to gut microflora and environment in addition to self-antigens through feedback network to maintain homeostasis [1–3] bridging innate and adaptive immune response. Thus, any chronic inflammation combined with compromised central tolerance can culminate into autoimmune disease [4]. However, autoimmune diseases have gender bias with prevalence in females owing to 'autoimmune X chromosome' and autoimmune infertility (AI) is no exception [5]. Concomitantly, reproductive autoimmune failure could result from an activated immune system or by anti-ovarian antibodies (AOA) alone as described in endometriosis patients [6]. Other reproductive disorders such as POI, polycystic ovary syndrome (PCOS), unexplained infertility, and repeatedly unsuccessful IVF attempts may be responsible for the pathophysiology of preeclampsia or spontaneous abortions and may also have presence of multiple autoantibodies (AAbs) [7–11].

Immune dysregulation is the cause of unexplained or idiopathic infertility in 20–30% of infertile couples [12]. AI is diagnosed when spontaneously synthesized antibodies bind or react with sperm/oocyte to prevent any one or several events: fertilization, acrosome reaction, capacitation or embryo implantation. Despite much research into organ specific biomarkers, no specific and sensitive biomarkers have been identified making detection of AI elusive. Organ-specific autoimmune disease gets treated using established protocols without sufficient consideration for fertility of women. Detection of AAbs mandates management of endometriosis, POI and other idiopathic infertility as an autoimmune disease with the treatment having adverse effects. This chapter will focus on AI, briefly in males but mainly in females, to include:

1. autoantigenic targets identified in female infertility with special emphasis on endometriosis and POI,

2. current understanding of effect of autoantibodies using animal models of disease,

3. including (AAbs) as diagnostic tools: current practices and

4. future research.

2. Male autoimmune infertility: anti-sperm antibodies (ASA)

Sperm are specialized haploid cells with autoantigenic and isoantigenic potential. Thus, ASA can be present in blood, semen, follicular fluid and cervicovaginal secretions affecting sperm movement, capacitation, fertilization and embryo implantation [13, 14]. ASA are far more frequent than oocyte antibodies.

In testis, the Sertoli cells through tight junctions form the impervious blood-testis barrier of two compartments: basal and adluminal. Basal compartment, which houses spermatogonia and young spermatocytes, is connected to vasculature through phagocytic Sertoli cells, which in turn act as antigen presenting cells to induce tolerance. The adluminal surface housing sperm undergoing meiosis and spermiogenesis is segregated from vasculature. Thus leakage of autoantigens from basal compartment can potentially generate ASAs. However, the exact mechanism of ASA generation is still unclear [13]. In some cases, Human Leucocyte Antigen system is associated with ASA and AI [15]. In 0.9–4% of normal fertile adult males as well as pre-pubertal boys, ASA are found in blood serum, seminal plasma, or directly attached to sperm surface indicating these to be NAbs generating confusion on their role in human infertility [16, 17].

Very few ASA are sperm specific [18] and never directed to multiple organs (except in animals). These can appear more frequently due to testicular failures: cryptorchidism, undescended testes, mobile testes and orchitis (especially due to infectious diseases such as mumps). Additionally, varicocele increases the risk of ASA production by two-fold [19]. The reduced testosterone levels due to altered Leydig cell function in undescended testes could theoretically result in reduced T regulatory cells and compromised central tolerance, however, exact mechanism is unclear. Elevated ASA could lead to low sperm count or low progressive motility. Hence, surgery at an early age, followed by steroid therapy to suppress immune reaction is recommended to prevent future infertility in cases with testicular failure.

ASA could be against carbohydrate moieties and sperm antigens example integral membrane proteins (exposed due to undescended testes) mainly through molecular mimicry. Natural ASA are reported in rodents due to sperm antigenic 'leak' to ensure immune tolerance. ASA are generally associated with genital tract infections. Vasectomy induces AAbs to antigens of mature human sperm [20, 21] with HLABw22 and A28 having increased predisposition post vasectomy [22]. Incidence reported is 61% pre- and 73–80% post-vasectomy. Antigens could be of either testicular or epididymal origin (epididymal maturation) with Abs directed to acrosome, equatorial and postacrosomal regions, tail midpiece and sperm nucleus. This could be due to sperm leakage in either the vas or cauda epididymis [21]. AutoAbs to FA-1 antigen (44%) and protamine (28%) seen post vasectomy in sera (none in seminal plasma) with prevalence of reduced fertilization rate *in vitro*. These were either of IgG, M or A subclass [23]. Post vasectomy ASA are seen only in serum while in seminal plasma and ejaculate post vasovasostomy. Fertile men with no ASA before vasovasostomy will show ASA that can affect sperm count [24, 25]. Further, there is no overlap of ASA between infertile men, post vasectomy [26] and post vasovasostomy. However, there are conflicting reports on their influence on pregnancy rate [27, 28]. **Table 1** enlists ASA in men with autoimmune infertility.

High titers of IgA-ASA found in seminal plasma of infertile men bind sperm head and impair fertilizing ability, the IgG elicit opsonization, and IgM from vaginal washings of vaginitis cases reduce fertilization by 44% [13]. ASAs directed to surface antigens are clinically relevant since they affect semen quality (not morphology or count) by any one of: premature acrosome reaction making the sperm moribund, sperm agglutination leading to impairment in cervical mucus penetration, opsonization through female genital tract via complement pathway.

ASA may aid sperm capacitation with no adverse effects on sperm-oocyte fusion. However, ASA binding outer acrosomal membrane proteins are washed away during procedure and do not affect IVF-intracytoplasmic sperm injection (IVF-ICSI) outcomes unlike those in females which are reported to reduce cleavage rate [47–49], with multiple autoantigenic targets necessary for AI [50].

Typically in women, the mucosal immunity protects entire reproductive tract up to Fallopian tubes against incoming sperm or any microbes. Thus vaginal and cervical secretions may contain ASA due to multiple semen exposures causing autoantigenicity to seminal fluid proteins. In rare cases of Human Seminal Plasma Allergy, first exposure can elicit antibodies [51] though it is not always associated with infertility [52, 53].

Autoantigen	Body fluid compartment	Function	Reference
Nuclear autoantigenic sperm protein (NASP) histone binding	Serum	Lowers fertilization rate	[29]
Protamines	Serum	–	[30]
DNA polymerase	Seminal plasma	–	[31]
YLP 12 peptide	Serum	acrosome reaction, union of sperm-oocyte	[32]
HSP70, 70-2 and 90	Serum	Acrosome reaction	[26]
Disulfide isomerase ER60	–	–	[26]
Sperm agglutination antigen-1 (SAGA-1)	–	–	[33]
Alpha enolase	Serum	–	[34]
Rab GDP-dissociation inhibitor beta		–	
Elongation factor 2		–	
Human G-phosphogluconate dehydrogenase, decarboxylating		–	
GAPDH-2		–	
L-Lactate dehydrogenase C chain		–	
ATP synthase beta chain mitochondrial precursor		–	
Proacrosin binding protein sp32	Seminal plasma	–	
CRISP-2		–	
ESP	Serum	Intra-acrosomal	[35]
SAMP 32			[36, 37]
SAMP14/ PH-20/hyaluronidase			[38]
AKAP 3		Fibrous sheath of the principal piece of the sperm tail	[39]
CABYR			[40–42]
RSP44		A radial spoke protein present in the axonemes of both sperm tail and cilia	[43]
FSP95		Fibrous sheath antigen	[44]
SLLP1		Intra-acrosomal protein	[44]
Zona pellucida			[8]
FSH			[45]
hESP	Serum	Sperm-egg binding and fusion	[46]

Table 1. List of autoantigens in men with autoimmune infertility.

ASA in females are of IgG, IgA and IgE subtypes in blood, lymph and cervical-vaginal mucus [50]. IgA antibodies in the cervical secretions can bind and agglutinate sperm with eventual clearance by circulating macrophages while the predominant IgG [54] can lead to opsonization and local clearance of antibody-antigen complexes. The uterus and Fallopian tubes are also protected by circulating macrophages and NK cells that clear the incoming sperm. Thus sperm coated with IgA-ASA are unaffected unlike those by IgG which are opsonized and cleared via macrophages. Both subtypes in the mucus individually affect fertilization alone while a combination significantly affects fertilization rate [55–58].

IgA alloantibodies to FSH are seen in some normal fertile women and can be produced during tolerance to partner antigens (sperm proteins and shared maternal antigens) through semen [59, 60]. Patients with increased intestinal permeability in bowel inflammatory disease show higher production of ASA through molecular mimicry or epitope sharing between intestinal microbes and spermatozoa [61]. An upregulated normal mucosal immune response could lead to the elevated levels of anti-FSH IgA antibodies in IVF patients. Another possible explanation could be a deficit in producing antibodies that neutralize anti-FSH immunoglobulins, which has been noted in patients who produce ASA [62]. These results together suggest that the elevated values of anti-FSH IgA in IVF patients could represent a failure in mucosal tolerance in the genital tract, which could be genetically determined [12] (**Table 2**). Enlists ASA detected in sera of women.

2.1. Diagnostic approaches and treatment modalities for couples with ASA

Presence of ASA in serum of seminal fluid binding to sperm outer membrane antigens and thereby altering fertilization rate are relevant, is inversely correlated with pregnancy and not a good indicator of pregnancy outcome. Testing for ASA is indicated for men with genitourinary infections (e.g., Chlamydia) or acquired genital tract obstructions. Nevertheless, these ASA may not always hinder pregnancy.

Sexually active homosexual individuals who have also undergone pelvic surgery should be advised to test for ASA [69]. Routine semen samples can be tested for sperm bound antibodies by IgG-mixed antiglobulin reaction (IgG-MAR [70]), immunobead test (IBT) [71] or sperm-MAR test [72]. However, none of the available diagnostic tests quantitate, are neither effective nor specific [73, 74]. Hence, instead of ineffective generalized immunosuppressive therapy IVF-ICSI should be considered [75–79].

Post vasovasostomy couples are advised IVF for pregnancy depending on body mass index and age which affect serum testosterone levels as well as ASA in men. In these cases, IVF may be beneficial only after testing for hypogonadism and serum testosterone levels [80]. ASA post

ASA	Body fluid compartment	Function	Reference
80 kDa protein	Serum	–	[63, 64]
BS 17		–	[65]
rSMP-B	–	–	[66]
Acrosin	Serum	Sperm-oocyte interaction	[67]
H-Y antigen		Secondary recurrent miscarriage	[68]

Table 2. List of autoantigenic targets against sera of women with ASA.

vasovasostomy can cause necrospermia and deteriorate sperm count hence IVF-ICSI using testicular sperm is an option [81].

3. Female autoimmune infertility

Women are prone to autoimmune diseases due to hormonally dictated cytokine and chemokine milieu [82] often leading to other autoimmune dysfunctions [83] including reproductive autoimmune failure. Gleicher and co-workers [6] postulated that endometriosis could be an autoimmune disease and studies from our lab show 30% prevalence [84]. Commonly seen serum AAbs are anti-phospholipid, anti-nuclear, anti-thyroid, anti-annexin V, anti-prothrombin, anti-laminin, anti-ZP (**Table 3** for entire list), with the high level of NK cells as the risk factors but not as those pathognomonic [85]. However, none of the AAb biomarkers tested were effective [86]. A recent study reported better sensitivity of 6 new biomarkers [87]. With detection of AAbs to steroid producing cells and thyroglobulin in cases with concomitant adrenal or thyroid disease in PCOS, it is now considered an autoimmune disease. However, anti-ovarian antibodies were reported in only one study [7, 88] with no clarity on their role in PCOS pathogenesis [89]. Organ-specific AAbs such as ovary, adrenal and thyroid (endocrine autoimmune) disease are reported to cause infertility due to premature ovarian insufficiency (POI) [90].

Both PCOS and endometriosis are also causative factors of POI. 40–60% women with endometriosis possess anti-ovarian Abs in addition to anti-endometrial Abs [103]. Several AAbs to non-organ specific targets are seen in women with unexplained infertility [104]. Further, 22% of patients with SLE show anti-corpus luteum antibodies and elevated FSH levels typical of POI [57] and 60% POI cases are of autoimmune origin [105, 106]. POI is typically detected late with both non-organ and organ-specific antibodies in conjunction with an autoimmune disease thus evading a specific and accurate biomarker for diagnosis and prognosis [107, 108]. Whether AAbs are causative of or a by-product of underlying disease is unclear.

Nevertheless, elaborate animal models of the disease as well as case studies have provided relevant data. Day three neonatal thymectomy mouse model showed that multi-organ autoimmune disease prevails. Immunization with a single antigen causes oophoritis alone while those to multiple antigens completely compromises ovarian function. Additionally, concomitant presence of the autoantigens was mandatory [109].

Efforts to identify target autoantigens based on discovery of an ovary specific autoantigen by ELISA, immunofluorescence or immunohistochemistry approach were unfruitful. This interference was due to non-specific reactivity of natural albumin antibodies [110]. Attempts to identify target autoantigens using sera and proteomics approach were fruitful enough to identify several somatic proteins: alpha actin, alpha actinin-4, heat shock proteins 70 and 90β in 30% of POI and 26% of IVF-ET failure cases [100, 111, 112]. Of these, 47% cases showed presence of AAbs to HSP90β. Reactivity of these antibodies was seen against several follicular components (**Table 4**). Note, besides oocyte the corpus luteum seems to be a major cellular target while HSP90β the molecular target contributing to early POI (bold and italics in **Table 4**) [111]. AAbs to MATER led to assuming it to be an ovary specific target [113] however, these

Autoantibodies	Compartment	Reference
Zona pellucida (ZP3, ZP2)	Peritoneal, follicular fluids, cervical-vaginal mucus	[50]
Anti-phospholipid	Cervical, serum	
Anti-cardiolipin	Serum	
Anti-HAL	Peritoneum	
Anti annexin 5		
FSH, β-subunit	Serum	[9, 12, 91–93]
17α-hydroxylase, desmolase (P450-side chain cleavage)		
3β-hydroxysteroid dehydrogenase		
21-hydroxylase		
Antinuclear autoantibodies (ANA)		
SMOOTH muscle autoantibodies (SMA)		
Anti-endometrial Abs		
Thyroid peroxidase		[94]
Alpha enolase		[95]
Aldehyde dehydrogenase		
Syntaxin 5		[86]
Cancer antigen 125 (CA125)		
Cancer antigen 19.9 (CA19.9)		
Serine/threonine-protein kinase (PDIK1L)		
Selenium binding protein 1		[96]
Heat-shock protein 90-β	Serum	[97]
LH receptor		[98, 99]
α-Actin	Serum	[100, 101]
α-Actinin-4		
HSPA5 (HSP70)		
Stomatin-like protein 2		[84, 87]
Tropomodulin 3 (TMOD3)		
Tropomyosin 3 (TPM3)		
Double stranded DNA	–	[89]
Angiotensin II type 1 receptor agonistic autoantibodies	Serum	[102]

Table 3. List of autoantigenic targets against sera of women with reproductive infertility.

AAbs were also seen in idiopathic hypoparathyroidism cases only in context of autoimmune polyendocrinopathy-candidiasis-ectodermal dystrophy syndrome [114].

Though a 75–90% accuracy was observed in ELISA assays using immunodominant epitopes from the identified targets, the AAbs were also present in normal population, highlighting the

Condition	Age at detection	Cellular target	Molecular target
POI	22	Oocyte, theca, *corpus luteum*	***90***
	33	Oocyte, *corpus luteum*	30
	38		45, ***90***
	24		***90***, 97
	33	Oocyte, theca, *corpus luteum*	97
	39	Oocyte, theca	***90***
	33	Theca	120
	38	Oocyte	***90***
	33	Ooplasm and nucleus of oocyte, theca	
	35	Oocyte	55
	36		97
	35	Oocyte of primordial follicle	70, 75
	32	Oocyte	70
	35	Granulosa, *corpus luteum*	30, 45
IVF-ET	29	Oocyte, *corpus luteum*	97
	28		120
	39		30, ***90***
	32	Oocyte	120
	34		50, 75, ***90***
	30	Oocyte, granulosa	80, 97
	28	Oocyte	120
	31	Theca	45, 97
	29	Oocyte	***90***, 120
	32		30, 50, ***90***
			90
	33	Oocyte	***90***, 97
	30	Zona pellucida	45

Table 4. List of antigens and cellular targets detected using sera of women with premature ovarian insufficiency (POI) and in vitro fertilization-embryo transfer (IVF-ET); compiled from [97].

fact that these were NAbs. These were also validated to induce aPOI in a mouse model. The immunodominant epitopes tested were able to induce POI and alter ovarian cytoarchitecture. Folliculogenesis was severely affected at each developmental stage with gross lack of mature Graafian follicles and a persistent corpus luteum [101].

AAbs to a single immunodominant epitope (EP6) HSP90β led to 9% dissociated oocyte-cumulus complexes, granulosa cells undergoing apoptosis, 48% empty follicles, and 12% degenerated follicles. These animals demonstrated significant pre- and post-implantation loss with concomitant decrease in fertility index along with an increased polymorphonuclear cell infiltration of the ovarian follicles. The infiltration may have contributed to generation of antibodies against the EP6 peptide [115, 116].

In normal physiological inflammatory processes like ovulation, follicular atresia, corpus luteum regression and tissue remodeling, the ovarian leukocytes like T cells and macrophages play an important role [117, 118]. Interestingly, NAbs especially, IgM play a role in clearing apoptotic cells, maintaining B cell homeostasis, inflammation, atherosclerosis and autoimmunity. Any drop in IgM levels is associated with ineffective clearance of apoptotic cells culminating into autoimmune disease. Alternatively, strong and persistent recognition of apoptotic cells by such NAbs may overactivate the immune system and cause chronic inflammation [3]. Corticosteroid treatment resolves the ensuing infertility [119]. However, there are no randomized controlled trials (RCT) to date. Our animal studies showed high dose corticosteroid was better able to rescue fertility in mice immunized with immunodominant epitopes of HSPA5 (**Table 5**). An interesting finding was the epitope spreading observed: AAbs to HSPA5 cross-react with immunodominant epitope (EP6) of HSP90β at high titer [120]. Thus, autoreactivity to HSP90β could have diagnostic and prognostic value.

Thyroid autoimmunity is commonly found with other systemic autoimmune diseases [121, 122] and is associated with anti-phospholipid syndrome (APS) due to anti-phospholipid antibodies [123] which in turn mediate recurrent miscarriages common to APS [124]. Thus women with thyroid autoimmunity and APS have greater risk of recurrent miscarriages mandating screening for anti-phospholipid antibodies. AAbs to ANA (12%), ANCA (20%), AECA (24%), ACLA (8%), anti-dsDNA (0%), β2 microglobulin (14%), and anti-HLA antibodies (10%) have been reported among Indian RSA patients [125]. This indicates that women with thyroiditis, endometriosis, SLE, APS also run the risk of repeated miscarriages.

At least 20–30% of POI cases have an additional autoimmune disorder [126] including several endocrinopathies, thyroid diseases, Addison's disease, rheumatoid arthritis and polyglandular

AutoAb target	Cellular target	Effect on estrus cycle	Delay in vaginal plug	Preimplantation loss	Fertility reduction	Effect of corticosteroid treatment
Alpha actinin-4	Ooplasm, theca and corpus luteum	Not determined	30%	24%	32%	44%
HSPA5	Ooplasm, granulosa, theca and corpus luteum		–	44%		
Alpha actin	Ooplasm, granulosa and theca,		30%	36.4%		
HSP90-beta (EP6)	Granulosa cells, developing embryo	Not significant	Not determined			
MATER/NALP5 (parathyroid autoantigen)	oocytes of later-stage small follicles	Not determined				

Table 5. Effect of autoantibodies on fertility and extent of rescue with corticosteroid therapy.

syndrome with greater prevalence of thyroid autoimmunity (14–27% at initial diagnosis) and thyroid peroxidase AAbs [127, 128]. At least 10% women with Addison's disease manifest AAbs to 21- or 17-hydroxylase and autoimmune oophoritis [129]. Thyroid peroxidase antibodies (TPO Abs) are also prevalent in PCOS cases. Thus, these along with HSP90β could be included in an antibody detection panel.

In women with endometriosis, use of biomarkers including CA-125 for diagnosis of endometriosis was prohibited [130, 131]. However as per recent guidelines, use of biomarkers has been recommended for both diagnosis and disease monitoring [132] and is still a researchable area. Anti-endometrial antibodies exist but their sensitivity and accuracy varies from 0 to 100% [131, 133, 134].

3.1. Treatment modalities and management of autoimmune infertility

Endometriosis management guidelines are valid for women with mild to moderate disease and do not recommend hormonal therapy for managing ovulation to improve fertility rate [135]. Despite reduction in ovarian function, one time laparoscopic operation to remove endometriosis and improve pregnancy rates is often recommended [136, 137]. Adjunctive hormonal therapy is prohibited pre- or post-surgery to improve pregnancy rates [138]. Intra uterine insemination along with controlled ovarian stimulation is recommended 6 months post-surgery since it shows similar pregnancy rates as that of women with unexplained infertility [139]. ART can also be recommended especially in cases of tubal factor or male factor infertility as controlled ovarian stimulation does not increase chances of recurrence of endometriosis after IVF/ICSI [140–143] however, it may not always be effective [144, 145].

POI seems to be an end-stage disease in women with an autoimmune disorder since it is detected at a late stage when the ovary has been substantially ravaged with little scope for fertility management. Thus treatment options for fertility management of women with POI are limited. Counseling for early marriage and pregnancy to complete the family is applicable only in case of early diagnosis or known familial origin. Other options include egg donation and IVF-ICSI or surrogacy. The women are administered corticosteroids in case of known autoimmune disease diagnosis and advised IVF-ICSI when AAb titers fall. However, this is not an option since it entails risk of osteoporosis and iatrogenic Cushing's syndrome [119]. In most cases, adoption is the only option along with psychological counseling and cardiovascular and bone health management of hypoestrogenism effects [146].

Additionally, there should be efforts to increase awareness among reproductive endocrinologists to recommend testing for undiagnosed autoimmune disease to couples on a case basis before embarking on ART-IVF [147].

4. Future research

Presence of AAbs is hallmark of autoimmune disease with no clarity on their role in disease pathogenesis and ensuing AI. With few exceptions these are not organ-specific indicating them

http://dx.doi.org/10.5772/intechopen.73899

to be NAbs [148–151]. Obtaining clarity on role of AAbs will guide further treatment modalities for patients with AI [93, 101, 152]. Global high dose immunosuppressive therapy seems to be the only effective option for autoimmune reproductive failure despite its shortcomings [153, 154].

Targeted interventional therapy by inducing antigen-specific tolerance is another option [155, 156]. Till such a time as a definitive therapy is available, pan autoimmune disease diagnostic panels can be designed using autoantigenic targets (recombinant proteins or peptides) such as β2-glycoprotein I and HSP90β (EP6) [151, 157–159] followed by management with corticosteroid therapy. A loss of reactivity to key autoantigens (predetermined to affect ovarian function) would serve as biomarkers to better manage immunosuppressant therapy.

5. Conclusion

The very lack of any organ-specific biomarker till date along with the preponderance of NAbs indicates that warped self-tolerance would lead to AI. AAbs in females alone appear to be significant in AI. Fertility studies need to be undertaken to gauge effect of such AAbs identified thus far and immunodominant epitopes gleaned could prove useful to design a pan autoimmune disease diagnostic peptide array to manage AI. Global immunosuppressant therapy and IVF-ICSI are the only current hope for such couples.

Acknowledgements

The work was co-funded by Indian Council of Medical Research and Dept. of Biotechnology, Govt. of India.

Conflict of interest

None.

Author details

Kaushiki M. Kadam[1]*, Purvi Mande[2] and Asmita Choudhury[2]

*Address all correspondence to: kaushikikadam@gmail.com

1 National Institute for Research in Reproductive Health, Indian Council of Medical Research, Mumbai, India

2 Department of Medicine, UMass Medical School, Worcester, MA, United States

References

[1] Poletaev A, Boura P. The immune system, natural autoantibodies and general homeostasis in health and disease. Hippokratia. 2011;**15**(4):295-298. PMCID: PMC3876841

[2] Siloşi I, Siloşi CA, Boldeanu MV, Cojocaru M, Biciuşcă V, Avrămescu CS, Cojocaru IM, Bogdan M, Folcuţi RM. The role of autoantibodies in health and disease. Romanian Journal of Morphology and Embryology. 2016;**57**(2):633-638. PMID: 27833954

[3] Panda S, Ding JL. Natural antibodies bridge innate and adaptive immunity. Journal of Immunology. 2015;**194**:13-20. DOI: https://doi.org/10.4049/jimmunol.1400844. PMID: 25527792

[4] Weiss G, Goldsmith LT, Taylor RN, Bellet D, Taylor HS. Inflammation in reproductive disorders. Reproductive Sciences. 2009;**16**(2):216-229. DOI: 10.1177/1933719108330087. PMID: 19208790

[5] Gleicher N, Kushnir VA, Barad DH. Prospectively assessing risk for premature ovarian senescence in young females: A new paradigm. Reproductive Biology and Endocrinology. 2015;**13**:34. DOI: 10.1186/s12958-015-0026-z. PMID: 25906823

[6] Gleicher N, El-Roeiy A, Confino E, Friberg J. Is endometriosis an autoimmune disease? Obstetrics & Gynecology. 1987;**70**(1):115-122. PMID: 3110710

[7] Fénichel P, Gobert B, Carré Y, Barbarino-Monnier P, Hiéronimus S. Polycystic ovary syndrome in autoimmune disease. Lancet. 1999;**353**(9171):2210. PMID: 10392989. DOI: 10.1016/S0140-6736(99)00256-1

[8] Forges T, Monnier-Barbarino P, Faure GC, Béné MC. Autoimmunity and antigenic targets in ovarian pathology. Human Reproduction Update. 2004;**10**(2):163-175. PMID: 15073145. DOI: 10.1093/humupd/dmh014

[9] Geva E, Amit A, Lerner-Geva L, Lessing JB. Autoimmunity and reproduction. Fertility and Sterility. 1997;**67**(4):599-611. PMID: 9093180

[10] Matarese G, de Placido G, Nikas Y, Alviggi C. Pathogenesis of endometriosis: Natural immunity dysfunction or autoimmune disease? Trends in Molecular Medicine. 2003; **9**(5):223-228. PMID: 12763528

[11] Reimand K, Talja I, Metsküla K, Kadastik Ü, Matt K, Uibo R. Autoantibody studies of female patients with reproductive failure. Journal of Reproductive Immunology. 2001; **51**(2):167-176. PMID: 11543855

[12] Haller-Kikkatalo K, Salumets A, Uibo R. Review on autoimmune reactions in female infertility: Antibodies to follicle stimulating hormone. Clinical & Developmental Immunology. 2012;**2012**:762541. PMID: 22007255. DOI: 10.1155/2012/762541

[13] Restrepo B, Cardona-Maya W. Antisperm antibodies and fertility association. Actas Urologicas Españolas. 2013;**37**(9):571-578. PMID: 23428233. DOI: 10.1016/j.acuro.2012.11.003

[14] Vazquez-Levin MH, Marín-Briggiler CI, Veaute C. Antisperm antibodies: Invaluable tools toward the identification of sperm proteins involved in fertilization. American Journal of Reproductive Immunology. 2014;**72**:206-218. PMID: 24863647. DOI: 10.1111/aji.12272

[15] Omu AE, Al-Qattan F, Ismail AA, Al-Taher S, Al-Busiri N. Relationship between unexplained infertility and human leukocyte antigens and expression of circulating autogeneic and allogeneic antisperm antibodies. Clinical and Experimental Obstetrics & Gynecology. 1999;**26**(3–4):199-202. PMID: 10668156

[16] Lu JC, Huang YF, Lu NQ. Antisperm immunity and infertility. Expert Review of Clinical Immunology. 2008;**4**(1):113-126. PMID: 20477591. DOI: 10.1586/1744666X.4.1.113

[17] Filippini A, Riccioli A, Padula F, Lauretti P, D'Alessio A, De Cesaris P, Gandini L, Lenzi A, Ziparo E. Control and impairment of immune privilege in the testis and in semen. Human Reproduction Update. 2001;**7**(5):444-449. PMID: 11556490

[18] Dörr H, Bohring C, Krause W. Are antisperm antibodies indeed sperm-specific? Andrologia. 2005;**37**:185-187. PMID: 16266397. DOI: 10.1111/j.1439-0272.2005.00675.x

[19] Bozhedomov VA, Lipatova NA, Rokhlikov IM, Alexeev RA, Ushakova IV, Sukhikh GT. Male fertility and varicocoele: Role of immune factors. Andrology. 2014;**2**:51-58. PMID: 24285668. DOI: 10.1111/j.2047-2927.2013.00160.x

[20] Phadke AM, Padukone K. Presence and significance of autoantibodies against spermatozoa in the blood of men with obstructed vas deferens. Journal of Reproduction and Fertility. 1964;**7**:163. PMID: 14139599

[21] Tung KSK. Human sperm antigens and antisperm antibodies. I. Studies on vasectomy patients. Clinical and Experimental Immunology. 1975;**20**:93-104. PMID: 1106922

[22] Law HY, Bodmer WF, Mathews JD, Skegg DC. The immune response to vasectomy and its relation to the HLA system. Tissue Antigens. 1979;**14**(2):115-139. PMID: 386565

[23] Naz RK, Deutsch J, Phillips TM, Menge AC, Fisch H. Sperm antibodies in vasectomized men and their effects on fertilization. Biology of Reproduction. 1989;**40**:163-173. PMID: 2804205

[24] Kay DJ, Clifton V, Taylor JS, Boettcher B. Anti-sperm antibodies and sperm profiles in re-anastomosed men. Reproduction, Fertility, and Development. 1993;**5**:135-139. PMID: 8234889

[25] Royle MG, Parslow JM, Kingscott MM, Wallace DM, Hendry WF. Reversal vasectomy: The effects of sperm antibodies on subsequent fertility. British Journal of Urology. 1981;**53**:654-659. PMID: 7032642

[26] Bohring C, Krause W. Differences in the antigen pattern recognized by antisperm antibodies in patients with infertility and vasectomy. The Journal of Urology. 2001;**166**(3):1178-1180. PMID: 11490318

[27] Meinertz H, Linnet L, Fogh-Andersen P, Hjort T. Antisperm antibodies and fertility after vasovasostomy: A follow-up study of 216 men. Fertility and Sterility. 1990;**54**(2):315-321. PMID: 2379630

[28] Lu WH, Liang XW, Gu YQ, Li H, Wu ZG, Chen ZW. The relationship between changes of serum antisperm antibodies before and post vasovasostomy and pregnancy rate. Zhonghua Nan Ke Xue. 2006;**12**(1):32-35, 38. PMID: 16483155

[29] Batova IN, Richardson RT, Widgren EE, O'Rand MG. Analysis of the autoimmune epitopes on human testicular NASP using recombinant and synthetic peptides. Clinical & Experimental Immunology. 2000;**121**(2):201-209. PMID: 10931132

[30] Samuel T, Linnet L, Rümke P. Post-vasectomy autoimmunity to protamines in relation to the formation of granulomas and sperm agglutinating antibodies. Clinical and Experimental Immunology. 1978;**33**(2):261-269. PMID: 102476

[31] Higgins PJ, Witkin SS, Bendich A. Inhibition of human seminal fluid DNA polymerase by an IgG fraction of seminal plasma from vasectomized men. Journal of Reproduction and Fertility. 1978;**54**(1):97-102. PMID: 101659

[32] Naz RK, Packianathan JLR. Antibodies to human sperm YLP12 peptide that is involved in egg binding inhibit human sperm capacitation/acrosome reaction. Archives of Andrology. 2000;**45**(3):227-232. PMID: 11111871

[33] Diekman AB, Norton EJ, Westbrook VA, Klotz KL, Naaby-Hansen S, Herr JC. Antisperm antibodies from infertile patients and their cognate sperm antigens: A review. Identity between SAGA-1, the H6-3C4 antigen, and CD52. American Journal of Reproductive Immunology. 2000;**43**(3):134-143. PMID: 10735589

[34] Domagała A, Pulido S, Kurpisz M, Herr JC. Application of proteomic methods for identification of sperm immunogenic antigens. Molecular Human Reproduction. 2007; **13**(7):437-444. PMID: 17507387. DOI: 10.1093/molehr/gam026

[35] Wolkowicz MJ, Shetty J, Westbrook A, Klotz K, Jayes F, Mandal A, Flickinger CJ, Herr JC. Equatorial segment protein defines a discrete acrosomal subcompartment persisting throughout acrosomal biogenesis. Biology of Reproduction. 2003;**69**:735-745. PMID: 12773409. DOI: 10.1095/biolreprod.103.016675

[36] Hao Z, Wolkowicz MJ, Shetty J, Klotz K, Bolling L, Sen B, Westbrook VA, Coonrod S, Flickinger CJ, Herr JC. SAMP32, a testis-specific, isoantigenic sperm acrosomal membrane-associated protein. Biology of Reproduction. 2002;**66**(3):735-744 11870081

[37] Rao J, Herr JC, Reddi PP, Wolkowicz MJ, Bush LA, Sherman NE, Black M, Flickinger CJ. Cloning and characterization of a novel sperm-associated isoantigen (E-3) with defensing and lectin-like motifs expressed in rat epididymis. Biology of Reproduction. 2003; **68**(1):290-301. PMID: 12493725

[38] Shetty J, Wolkowicz MJ, Digilio LC, Klotz KL, Jayes FL, Diekman AB, Westbrook VA, Farris EM, Hao Z, Coonrod SA, Flickinger CJ, Herr JC. SAMP14, a novel, acrosomal

membrane-associated, glycosylphosphatidylinositol-anchored member of the Ly-6/urokinase-type plasminogen activator receptor superfamily with a role in sperm-egg interaction. The Journal of Biological Chemistry. 2003;**278**(33):30506-30515. PMID: 12788941

[39] Mandal A, Naaby-Hansen S, Wolkowicz MJ, Klotz K, Shetty J, Retief JD, Coonrod SA, Kinter M, Sherman N, Cesar F, Flickinger CJ, Herr JC. FSP95, a testis-specific 95-kilodalton fibrous sheath antigen that undergoes tyrosine phosphorylation in capacitated human spermatozoa. Biology of Reproduction. 1999 Nov;**61**(5):1184-1197. PMID: 10529264

[40] Naaby-Hansen S, Mandal A, Wolkowicz MJ, Sen B, Westbrook VA, Shetty J, Coonrod SA, Klotz KL, Kim YH, Bush LA, Flickinger CJ, Herr JC. CABYR, a novel calcium-binding tyrosine phosphorylation-regulated fibrous sheath protein involved in capacitation. Developmental Biology. 2002;**242**(2):236-254. PMID: 11820818

[41] Sen B, Mandal A, Wolkowicz MJ, Kim YH, Reddi PP, Shetty J, Bush LA, Flickinger CJ, Herr JC. Splicing in murine CABYR and its genomic structure. Gene. 2003;**310**:67-78. PMID: 12801634

[42] Kim YH, Jha KN, Mandal A, Vanage G, Farris E, Snow PL, Klotz K, Naaby-Hansen S, Flickinger CJ, Herr JC. Translation and assembly of CABYR coding region B in fibrous sheath and restriction of calcium binding to coding region A. Developmental Biology. 2005;**286**(1):46-56. PMID: 16139264

[43] Shetty J, Klotz KL, Wolkowicz MJ, Flickinger CJ, Herr JC. Radial spoke protein 44 (human meichroacidin) is an axonemal alloantigen of sperm and cilia. Gene. 2007; **396**(1):93-107. PMID: 17451891. DOI: 10.1016/j.gene.2007.02.031

[44] Mandal A, Klotz KL, Shetty J, Jayes FL, Wolkowicz MJ, Bolling LC, Coonrod SA, Black MB, Diekman AB, Haystead TA, Flickinger CJ, Herr JC. SLLP1, a unique, intra-acrosomal, non-bacteriolytic, c lysozyme-like protein of human spermatozoa. Biology of Reproduction. 2003;**68**(5):1525-1537. PMID: 12606493

[45] Westhoff WE, Slootstra JW, Puijk WC, Kuperus D, Flinterman JF, Schaaper WM, Oonk HB, Meloen RH. Detection of epitopes on follicle-stimulating hormone and FSH antiserum-induced suppression of bioactivity of follicle stimulating hormone and luteinizing hormone. Journal of Reproductive Immunology. 1996;**30**(2–3):133-149. PMID: 8816329

[46] Wolkowicz MJ, Digilio L, Klotz K, Shetty J, Flickinger CJ, Herr JC. Equatorial segment protein (ESP) is a human alloantigen involved in sperm-egg binding and fusion. Journal of Andrology. 2008;**29**(3):272-282. PMID: 17978344

[47] Francavilla F, Santucci R, Barbonetti A, Francavilla S. Naturally-occurring antisperm antibodies in men: interference with fertility and clinical implications. An update. Frontiers in Bioscience. 2007;**12**:2890-2911. PMID: 17485267

[48] Mandelbaum SL, Diamond MP, AH DC. Relationship of antisperm antibodies to oocyte fertilization in in vitro fertilization-embryo transfer. Fertility and Sterility. 1987;**47**:644-651. PMID: 3552746

[49] Tian X, Zhang L, Wu Y, Yang C, Liu P. Relationship between serum antisperm antibodies and anticardiolipin antibodies and clinical pregnancy outcome in an in vitro fertilization and embryo transfer program. Chinese Medical Journal. 1999;**112**(1):34-36. PMID: 11593637

[50] Brázdová A, Senechal H, Peltre G, Poncet P. Immune aspects of female infertility. International Journal of Fertility & Sterility. 2016;**10**(1):1-10. PMID: 27123194

[51] James DW. Pernicious vomiting of pregnancy due to sensitivity to semen. Western Journal of Surgery, Obstetrics, and Gynecology. 1945;**53**:380-382

[52] Ebo DG, Stevens W, Bridts C, De Clerck L, Bernstein I. Human seminal plasma anaphylaxis (HSPA): Case report and literature review. Allergy. 1995;**50**:747-750. PMID: 8546271

[53] Weidinger S, Ring J, Köhn F. IgE-mediated allergy against human seminal plasma. Chemical Immunology and Allergy. 2005;**88**:128-138. PMID: 16129942. DOI: 10.1159/000087830

[54] Johansson M, Lycke N. Immunology of the human genital tract. Current Opinion in Infectious Diseases. 2003;**16**:43-49. PMID: 12821829

[55] Clarke GN, Lopata A, McBain JC, Baker HW, Johnston WI. Effect of sperm antibodies in males on human in vitro fertilization (IVF). American Journal of Reproductive Immunology and Microbiology. 1985;**8**:62-66. PMID: 4025668

[56] Matson PL, Junk SM, Spittle JW, Yovich JL. Effect of antispermatozoal antibodies in seminal plasma upon spermatozoal function. International Journal of Andrology. 1988; **11**:101-106. PMID: 3286524

[57] Junk SM, Matson PL, Yovich JM, Bootsma B, Yovich JL. The fertilization of human oocytes by spermatozoa from men with antispermatozoal antibodies in semen. Journal of In Vitro Fertilization and Embryo Transfer. 1986;**3**:350-352. PMID: 3805851

[58] de Almeida M, Gazagne I, Jeulin C, Herry M, Belaisch-Allart J, Frydman R, Jouannet P, Testart J. In vitro processing of sperm with auto-antibodies and in-vitro fertilization results. Human Reproduction. 1989;**4**:49-53. PMID: 2708503

[59] Hegde UC, Ranpura S, D'Souza S, Raghavan VP. Immunoregulatory pathways in pregnancy. Indian Journal of Biochemistry & Biophysics. 2001;**38**(4):207-219. PMID: 11811615

[60] Luboshitzky R, Kaplan-Zverling M, Shen-Orr Z, Nave R, Herer P. Seminal plasma androgen/oestrogen balance in infertile men. International Journal of Andrology. 2002; **25**(6):345-351. PMID: 12406366

[61] Dimitrova D, Kalaydjiev S, Mendizova A, Piryova E, Nakov L. Circulating antibodies to human spermatozoa in patients with ulcerative colitis. Fertility and Sterility. 2005;**84**(5): 1533-1535. PMID: 16275264. DOI: 10.1016/j.fertnstert.2005.05.041

[62] Naz RK, Ahmad K, Menge AC. Anti-idiotypic antibodies to sperm in sera of fertile women that neutralize antisperm antibodies. The Journal of Clinical Investigation. 1993;**92**(5):2331-2338. PMID: 8227348. DOI: 10.1172/JCI116837

[63] Bandivdekar AH, Gopalkrishnan K, Garde SV, Fernandez PX, Moodbidri SB, Sheth AR, Koide SS. Antifertility effect in rats actively immunized with 80kDa human semen glycoprotein. Indian Journal of Experimental Biology. 1992;**30**:1017-1023. PMID: 1293024

[64] Bandivdekar AH, Vernekar VJ, Moodbidri SB, Koide SS. Characterization of 80 kDa human sperm antigen responsible for immunoinfertility. American Journal of Reproductive Immunology. 2001;**45**(1):28-34. PMID: 11211944

[65] Wei SG, Wang LF, Miao SY, Zong SD, Koide SS. Fertility studies with antisperm antibodies. Archives of Andrology. 1994;**32**(3):251-262. PMID: 8074581

[66] Koide SS, Wang L, Kamada M. Antisperm antibodies associated with infertility: Properties and encoding genes of target antigens. Proceedings of the Society for Experimental Biology and Medicine. 2000;**224**:123-132. PMID: 10865226

[67] Veaute C, Furlong LI, Bronson R, Harris JD, Vazquez-Levin MH. Acrosin antibodies and infertility. I. Detection of antibodies towards proacrosin/acrosin in women consulting for infertility and evaluation of their effects upon the sperm protease activities. Fertility and Sterility. 2009;**91**(4):1245-1255. PMID: 18439585. DOI: 10.1016/j.fertnstert.2007.12.072

[68] Nielsen HS, Wu F, Aghai Z, Steffensen R, van Halteren AG, Spierings E, Christiansen OB, Miklos D, Goulmy E. H-Y antibody titers are increased in unexplained secondary recurrent miscarriage patients and associated with low male : Female ratio in subsequent live births. Human Reproduction. 2010;**25**(11):2745-2752. PMID: 20823116. DOI: 10.1093/humrep/deq242

[69] Marshburn PB, Kutteh WH. The role of antisperm antibodies in infertility. Fertility and Sterility. 1994;**61**:799-811. PMID: 8174713

[70] Jager S, Kremer J, van Slochteren-Draaisma T. A simple method of screening for antisperm antibodies in the human male: Detection of spermatozoan surface IgG with the direct mixed agglutination reaction carried out on untreated fresh human semen. International Journal of Fertility. 1978;**23**:12-21 30704

[71] Bronson R, Cooper G, Rosenfeld D. Membrane bound sperm-specific antibodies: Their role in infertility. In: Vogel H, Jagiello G, editors. Bioregulators in Reproduction. New York: Academic Press; 1981. pp. 521-527

[72] Comhaire FH, Hinting A, Vermeulen L, Schoonjans F, Goethals I. Evaluation of the direct and indirect mixed antiglobulin reaction with latex particles for the diagnosis of immunological infertility. International Journal of Andrology. 1987;**11**:37-44. PMID: 3258588

[73] Nikolaeva MA, Kulakov VI, Korotkova IV, Golubeva EL, Kuyavskaya DV, Sukhikh GT. Antisperm antibodies detection by flow cytometry is affected by aggregation of antigen-antibody complexes on the surface of spermatozoa. Human Reproduction. 2000;**15**(12): 2545-2553. PMID: 11098024

[74] Hjort T. Antisperm antibodies. Antisperm antibodies and infertility: An unsolvable question? Human Reproduction. 1999;**14**:2423-2426. PMID: 10527960

[75] Kamischke A, Nieschlag E. Analysis of medical treatment of male infertility. Human Reproduction. 1999;**14**(Suppl 1):1-23. PMID: 10573021

[76] Nagy ZP, Aragona C, Greco E. Results of ICSI in the treatment of male immunological infertility. Andrologia. 1999;**31**:316-317. PMID: 10526648

[77] Check ML, Check JH, Katsoff D, Summers-Chase D. ICSI as an effective therapy for male factor with antisperm antibodies. Archives of Andrology. 2000;**45**:125-130. PMID: 11111859

[78] Mardesic T, Ulcova-Gallova Z, Huttelova R, Muller P, Voboril J, Mikova M, Hulvert J. The influence of different types of antibodies on in vitro fertilization results. American Journal of Reproductive Immunology. 2000;**43**:1-5. PMID: 10698033

[79] Lombardo F, Gandini L, Dondero F, Lenzi A. Antisperm immunity in natural and assisted reproduction. Human Reproduction Update. 2001;**7**:450-456. PMID: 11556491

[80] Hinz S, Rais-Bahrami S, Kempkensteffen C, Weiske WH, Miller K, Magheli A. Effect of obesity on sex hormone levels, antisperm antibodies, and fertility after vasectomy reversal. Urology. 2010;**76**(4):851-856. DOI: 10.1016/j.urology.2010.01.055. PMID: 20430424

[81] Chavez-Badiola A, Drakeley AJ, Finney V, Sajjad Y, Lewis-Jones DI. Necrospermia, antisperm antibodies, and vasectomy. Fertility and Sterility. 2008;**89**(3):723.e5-723.e7. PMID: 17612533. DOI: 10.1016/j.fertnstert.2007.04.007

[82] Smith-Bouvier DL, Divekar AA, Sasidhar M, Du S, Tiwari-Woodruff SK, King JK, Arnold AP, Singh RR, Voskuhl RR. A role for sex chromosome complement in the female bias in autoimmune disease. The Journal of Experimental Medicine. 2008;**205**(5): 1099-1108. PMID: 18443225. DOI: 10.1084/jem.20070850

[83] Tuohy VK, Kinkel RP. Epitope spreading: A mechanism for progression of autoimmune disease. Archivum Immunologiae et Therapiae Experimentalis (Warsz). 2000;**48**(5):347-351. PMID: 11140461

[84] Gajbhiye R, Suryawanshi A, Khan S, Meherji P, Warty N, Raut V, Chehna N, Khole V. Multiple endometrial antigens are targeted in autoimmune endometriosis. Reproductive Biomedicine Online. 2008;**16**(6):817-824. PMID: 18549691

[85] Gleicher N, Barad D. Unexplained infertility: Does it really exist? Human Reproduction. 2006;**21**(8):1951-1955. PMID: 16684842. DOI: 10.1093/humrep/del135

[86] Nisenblat V, Bossuyt PM, Shaikh R, Farquhar C, Jordan V, Scheffers CS, Mol BW, Johnson N, Hull ML. Blood biomarkers for the non-invasive diagnosis of endometriosis. Cochrane Database of Systematic Reviews. 2016;**1**(5):CD012179. PMID: 27132058. DOI: 10.1002/14651858.CD012179

[87] Gajbhiye R, Bendigeri T, Ghuge A, Bhusane K, Begum S, Warty N, Sawant R, Padte K, Humane A, Dasmahapatra P, Chauhan A, Khan S. Panel of autoimmune markers for noninvasive diagnosis of minimal-mild endometriosis. Reproductive Sciences. 2017; **24**(3):413-420. PMID: 27485360. DOI: 10.1177/1933719116657190

[88] Mobeen H, Afzal N, Kashif M. Polycystic ovary syndrome may be an autoimmune disorder. Scientifica (Cairo). 2016;**2016**:4071735. PMID: 27274883. DOI: 10.1155/2016/4071735

[89] Petrikova J, Lazurova I, Dravecka I, Vrbikova J, Kozakova D, Figurova J, Vaczy Z, Rosocha J. The prevalence of non-organ specific and thyroid autoimmunity in patients with polycystic ovary syndrome. Biomedical Papers of the Medical Faculty of the University Palacky, Olomouc, Czech Republic. 2015;**159**(2):302-306. PMID: 25485530. DOI: 10.5507/bp.2014.062

[90] Hoek A, Schoemaker J, Drexhage HA. Premature ovarian failure and ovarian autoimmunity. Endocrine Reviews. 1997 Feb;**18**(1):107-134 Review. PMID: 9034788

[91] Mathur S, Peress MR, Williamson HO. Autoimmunity to endometrium and ovary in endometriosis. Clinical and Experimental Immunology. 1982;**50**(2):259-266. PMID: 6759000

[92] Ulcová-Gallová Z, Bouse V, Svábek L, Turek J, Rokyta Z. Endometriosis in reproductive immunology. American Journal of Reproductive Immunology. 2002;**47**(5):269-274. PMID: 12148541

[93] Zou SH, Yang ZZ, Zhang P, Song DP, Li B, Wu RY, Cong X. Autoimmune disorders affect the in vitro fertilization outcome in infertile women. Zhonghua Nan Ke Xue. 2008;**14**(4):343-346. PMID: 18481429

[94] Poppe K, Glinoer D, Van Steirteghem A, Tournaye H, Devroey P, Schiettecatte J, Velkeniers B. Thyroid dysfunction and autoimmunity in infertile women. Thyroid. 2002;**12**(11):997-1001. PMID: 12490077. DOI: 10.1089/105072502320908330

[95] Sarapik A, Haller-Kikkatalo K, Utt M, Teesalu K, Salumets A, Uibo R. Serum anti-endometrial antibodies in infertile women—Potential risk factor for implantation failure. American Journal of Reproductive Immunology. 2010;**63**(5):349-357. PMID: 20132165. DOI: 10.1111/j.1600-0897.2010.00808.x

[96] Yu-Rice Y, Edassery SL, Urban N, Hellstrom I, Hellstrom KE, Deng Y, Li Y, Luborsky JL. Selenium-binding protein 1 (SBP1) autoantibodies in ovarian disorders and ovarian cancer. Reproduction. 2017;**153**:277-284. PMID: 27965399. DOI: 10.1530/REP-16-0265

[97] Pires ES, Meherji PK, Vaidya RR, Parikh FR, Ghosalkar MN, Khole VV. Specific and sensitive immunoassays detect multiple anti-ovarian antibodies in women with infertility. The Journal of Histochemistry and Cytochemistry. 2007;**55**(12):1181-1190. PMID: 17652265. DOI: 10.1369/jhc.7A7259.2007

[98] Wheatcroft NJ, Toogood AA, Li TC, Cooke ID, Weetman AP. Detection of antibodies to ovarian antigens in women with premature ovarian failure. Clinical and Experimental Immunology. 1994;**96**(1):122-128. PMID: 8149656

[99] Moncayo H, Moncayo R, Benz R, Wolf A, Lauritzen C. Ovarian failure and autoimmunity. Detection of autoantibodies directed against both the unoccupied luteinizing hormone/human chorionic gonadotropin receptor and the hormone-receptor complex of

ovine corpus luteum. The Journal of Clinical Investigation. 1989;**84**(6):1857-1865. PMID: 2592563. DOI: 10.1172/JCI114372

[100] Mande PV, Parikh FR, Hinduja I, Zaveri K, Vaidya R, Gajbhiye R, Khole VV. Identification and validation of candidate biomarkers involved in human ovarian autoimmunity. Reproductive Biomedicine Online. 2011;**23**(4):471-483. PMID: 21890413. DOI: 10.1016/j.rbmo.2011.06.013

[101] Mande PV, Thomas S, Khan S, Jadhav S, Khole VV. Immunization with ovarian autoantigens leads to reduced fertility in mice following follicular dysfunction. Reproduction. 2012;**143**(3):309-323. PMID: 22143970. DOI: 10.1530/REP-11-0221

[102] Kobayashi Y, Yamamoto T, Chishima F, Takahashi H, Suzuki M. Autoantibodies isolated from patients with preeclampsia induce soluble endoglin production from trophoblast cells via interactions with angiotensin II type 1 receptor. American Journal of Reproductive Immunology. 2015;**73**:285-291. PMID: 25376533. DOI: 10.1111/aji.12340

[103] Komorowska B. Autoimmune premature ovarian failure. Prz Menopauzalny. 2016;**15, 4**: 210-214. PMID: 28250725. DOI: 10.5114/pm.2016.65666

[104] Cervera R, Balasch J. Bidirectional effects on autoimmunity and reproduction. Human Reproduction Update. 2008;**14**(4):359-366. PMID: 18499707. DOI: 10.1093/humupd/dmn013

[105] Luborsky JL, Visintin I, Boyers S, et al. Ovarian antibodies detected by immobilized antigen immunoassay in patients with premature ovarian failure. The Journal of Clinical Endocrinology and Metabolism. 1990;**70**:69-75. PMID: 2104631. DOI: 10.1210/jcem-70-1-69

[106] Lebovic DI, Naz R. Premature ovarian failure: Think 'autoimmune disorder'. Sexuality, Reproduction & Menopause. 2004;**2**(4):230-233

[107] Betterle C, Dal Pra C, Mantero F, Zanchetta R. Autoimmune adrenal insufficiency and autoimmune polyendocrine syndromes: Autoantibodies, autoantigens, and their applicability in diagnosis and disease prediction. Endocrine Reviews. 2002;**23**:327-364. PMID: 12050123. DOI: 10.1210/edrv.23.3.0466

[108] Ebrahimi M, Akbari Asbagh F. Pathogenesis and causes of premature ovarian failure: An update. International Journal of Fertility & Sterility. 2011;**5**:54-65. PMID: 24963360

[109] Bagavant H, Thompson C, Ohno K, Setiady Y, Tung KS. Differential effect of neonatal thymectomy on systemic and organ-specific autoimmune disease. International Immunology. 2002;**14**(12):1397-1406. PMID: 12456587

[110] Pires ES, Parte PP, Meherji PK, Khan SA, Khole VV. Naturally occurring anti-albumin antibodies are responsible for false positivity in diagnosis of autoimmune premature ovarian failure. The Journal of Histochemistry and Cytochemistry. 2006 Apr;**54**(4):397-405 Epub 2005 Nov 14. PMID: 16286665

[111] Pires ES, Khole VV. A block in the road to fertility: Autoantibodies to heat-shock protein 90-beta in human ovarian autoimmunity. Fertility and Sterility. 2009 Oct;**92**(4):1395-1409. DOI: 10.1016/j.fertnstert.2008.08.068 Epub 2008 Nov 19. PMID: 19022436

[112] Pires ES, Choudhury AK, Idicula-Thomas S, Khole VV. Anti-HSP90 autoantibodies in sera of infertile women identify a dominant, conserved epitope EP6 (380-389) of HSP90 beta protein. Reproductive Biology and Endocrinology. 2011;**9**:16. DOI: 10.1186/1477-7827-9-16. PMID: 21272367

[113] Tong ZB, Nelson LM. A mouse gene encoding an oocyte antigen associated with autoimmune premature ovarian failure. Endocrinology. 1999;**140**:3720-3726. PMID: 10433232. DOI: 10.1210/endo.140.8.6911

[114] Tomar N, Kaushal E, Das M, Gupta N, Betterle C, Goswami R. Prevalence and significance of NALP5 autoantibodies in patients with idiopathic hypoparathyroidism. The Journal of Clinical Endocrinology and Metabolism. 2012;**97**(4):1219-1226. PMID: 22278434. DOI: 10.1210/jc.2011-3093

[115] Choudhury A, Khole VV. HSP90 antibodies: A detrimental factor responsible for ovarian dysfunction. American Journal of Reproductive Immunology. 2013;**70**(5):372-385. PMID: 23662883. DOI: 10.1111/aji.12136

[116] Choudhury A, Khole VV. Immune-mediated destruction of ovarian follicles associated with the presence of HSP90 antibodies. Molecular Reproduction and Development. 2015;**82**(2):81-89. PMID: 25653208. DOI: 10.1002/mrd.22428

[117] Bukulmez O, Arici A. Leukocytes in ovarian function. Human Reproduction Update. 2000;**6**:1-15. PMID: 10711825

[118] Wu R, Van der Hoek KH, Ryan NK, Norman RJ, Robker RL. Macrophage contributions to ovarian function. Human Reproduction Update. 2004;**10**:119-133. PMID: 15073142. DOI: 10.1093/humupd/dmh011

[119] Kalantaridou SN, Braddock DT, Patronas NJ, Nelson LM. Treatment of autoimmune premature ovarian failure. Human Reproduction. 1999;**14**(7):1777-1782. PMID: 10402388

[120] Kadam KM, Mande PV, Gawas N, Ahire S, Khole VV. Autoantibodies to heat-shock protein, HSPA5, and epitope spreading: High-dose dexamethasone therapy rescues ovarian function in experimental autoimmune ovarian insufficiency mouse model. American Journal of Reproductive Immunology. 2016;**75**:580-593. PMID: 26840828. DOI: 10.1111/aji.12494

[121] Antonelli A, Ferrari SM, Corrado A, Di Domenicantonio A, Fallahi P. Autoimmune thyroid disorders. Autoimmunity Reviews. 2015;**14**(2):174-180. PMID: 25461470. DOI: 10.1016/j.autrev.2014.10.016

[122] Robazzi TC, Adan LF. Autoimmune thyroid disease in patients with rheumatic diseases. Revista Brasileira de Reumatologia. 2012;**52**(3):417-430. PMID: 22641595

[123] Versini M. Thyroid autoimmunity and antiphospholipid syndrome: Not such a trivial association. Frontiers in Endocrinology. 2017;**8**:175. PMID: 28785243. DOI: 10.3389/fendo.2017.00175

[124] Souza SS, Ferriani RA, Santos CM, Voltarelli JC. Immunological evaluation of patients with recurrent abortion. Journal of Reproductive Immunology. 2002;**56**:111-121. PMID: 12106887

[125] Shankarkumar U, Pradhan VD, Patwardhan MM, Shankarkumar A, Ghosh K. Autoantibody profile and other immunological parameters in recurrent spontaneous abortion patients. Nigerian Medical Journal. 2011;**52**(3):163-166. PMCID: PMC3213746. DOI: 10.4103/0300-1652.86126

[126] Petríková J, Lazúrová I. Ovarian failure and polycystic ovary syndrome. Autoimmunity Reviews. 2012;**11**(6–7):A471-A478. PMID: 22154711. DOI: 10.1016/j.autrev.2011.11.010

[127] Goswami R, Marwaha RK, Goswami D, Gupta N, Ray D, Tomar N, Singh S. Prevalence of thyroid autoimmunity in sporadic idiopathic hypoparathyroidism in comparison to type 1 diabetes and premature ovarian failure. Journal of Clinical Endocrinology and Metabolism. 2006;**91**(11):4256-4259. PMID: 16895958. DOI: 10.1210/jc.2006-1005

[128] Nelson LM. Clinical practice. Primary ovarian insufficiency. The New England Journal of Medicine. 2009;**360**:606-614. PMCID: PMC2762081. DOI: 10.1056/NEJMcp0808697

[129] Kifor O, Moore FD Jr, Delaney M, Garber J, Hendy GN, Butters R, Gao P, Cantor TL, Kifor I, Brown EM, Wysolmerski J. A syndrome of hypocalciuric hypercalcemia caused by autoantibodies directed at the calcium-sensing receptor. The Journal of Clinical Endocrinology and Metabolism. 2003;**88**(1):60-72. PMID: 12519831. DOI: 10.1210/jc.2002-020249

[130] Mol BW, Bayram N, Lijmer JG, Wiegerinck MA, Bongers MY, van der Veen F, Bossuyt PM. The performance of CA-125 measurement in the detection of endometriosis: A meta-analysis. Fertility and Sterility. 1998;**70**:1101-1108. PMID: 9848302

[131] May KE, Conduit-Hulbert SA, Villar J, Kirtley S, Kennedy SH, Becker CM. Peripheral biomarkers of endometriosis: A systematic review. Human Reproduction Update. 2010; **16**:651-674. PMID: 20462942. DOI: 10.1093/humupd/dmq009

[132] Dunselman GAJ, Vermeulen N, Becker C, Calhaz-Jorge C, D'Hooghe T, De Bie B, Heikinheimo O, Horne AW, Kiesel L, Nap A, Prentice A, Saridogan E, Soriano D, Nelen W. ESHRE guideline: Management of women with endometriosis. Human Reproduction. 2014;**29**(3):400-412. PMID: 24435778. DOI: 10.1093/humrep/det457

[133] May KE, Villar J, Kirtley S, Kennedy SH, Becker CM. Endometrial alterations in endometriosis: A systematic review of putative biomarkers. Human Reproduction Update. 2011;**17**(5):637-653. PMID: 21672902. DOI: 10.1093/humupd/dmr013

[134] Fassbender A, Burney RO, DF O, D'Hooghe T, Giudice L. Update on biomarkers for the detection of endometriosis. BioMed Research International. 2015;**2015**:130854. PMID: 26240814. DOI: 10.1155/2015/130854

[135] Hughes E, Brown J, Collins JJ, Farquhar C, Fedorkow DM, Vandekerckhove P. Ovulation suppression for endometriosis. Cochrane Database of Systematic Reviews. 2007: CD000155. PMID: 17636607. DOI: 10.1002/14651858.CD000155.pub2

[136] Nowroozi K, Chase JS, Check JH, Wu CH. The importance of laparoscopic coagulation of mild endometriosis in infertile women. International Journal of Fertility. 1987;**32**:442-444. PMID: 2891631

[137] Jacobson TZ, Duffy JM, Barlow D, Farquhar C, Koninckx PR, Olive D. Laparoscopic surgery for subfertility associated with endometriosis. Cochrane Database of Systematic Reviews. 2010:CD001398. PMID: 20091519. DOI: 10.1002/14651858.CD001398.pub2

[138] Yap C, Furness S, Farquhar C. Pre and post-operative medical therapy for endometriosis surgery. Cochrane Database of Systematic Reviews. 2004:CD003678. PMID: 15266496. DOI: 10.1002/14651858.CD003678.pub2

[139] Werbrouck E, Spiessens C, Meuleman C, D'Hooghe T. No difference in cycle pregnancy rate and in cumulative live-birth rate between women with surgically treated minimal to mild endometriosis and women with unexplained infertility after controlled ovarian hyperstimulation and intrauterine insemination. Fertility and Sterility. 2006;**86**:566-571. PMID: 16952506. DOI: 10.1016/j.fertnstert.2006.01.044

[140] D'Hooghe TM, Denys B, Spiessens C, Meuleman C, Debrock S. Is the endometriosis recurrence rate increased after ovarian hyperstimulation? Fertility and Sterility. 2006;**86**: 283-290. PMID: 16753162. DOI: 10.1016/j.fertnstert.2006.01.016

[141] Benaglia L, Somigliana E, Vercellini P, Benedetti F, Iemmello R, Vighi V, Santi G, Ragni G. The impact of IVF procedures on endometriosis recurrence. European Journal of Obstetrics, Gynecology, and Reproductive Biology. 2010;**148**:49-52. PMID: 19800161. DOI: 10.1016/j.ejogrb.2009.09.007

[142] Benaglia L, Somigliana E, Santi G, Scarduelli C, Ragni G, Fedele L. IVF and endometriosis-related symptom progression: Insights from a prospective study. Human Reproduction. 2011;**26**:2368-2372. PMID: 21715451. DOI: 10.1093/humrep/der208

[143] Coccia ME, Rizzello F, Gianfranco S. Does controlled ovarian hyperstimulation in women with a history of endometriosis influence recurrence rate? Journal of Women's Health (2002). 2010;**19**:2063-2069. PMID: 20831441. DOI: 10.1089/jwh.2009.1914

[144] Bianchi PH, Pereira RM, Zanatta A, Alegretti JR, Motta EL, Serafini PC. Extensive excision of deep infiltrative endometriosis before in vitro fertilization significantly improves pregnancy rates. Journal of Minimally Invasive Gynecology. 2009;**16**(2):174-180. PMID: 19249705. DOI: 10.1016/j.jmig.2008.12.009

[145] Papaleo E, Ottolina J, Vigano P, Brigante C, Marsiglio E, De Michele F, Candiani M. Deep pelvic endometriosis negatively affects ovarian reserve and the number of oocytes retrieved for in vitro fertilization. Acta Obstetricia et Gynecologica Scandinavica. 2011; **90**:878-884. PMID: 21542809. DOI: 10.1111/j.1600-0412.2011.01161.x

[146] Webber L, Davies M, Anderson R, Bartlett J, Braat D, Cartwright B, Cifkova R, De Muinck Keizer-Schrama S, Hogervorst E, Janse F, Liao L, Vlaisavljevic V, Zillikens C, Vermeulen N. ESHRE guideline: Management of women with premature ovarian insufficiency. Human Reproduction. 2016;**31**(5):926-937. PMID: 27008889. DOI: 10.1093/humrep/dew027

[147] Klonoff-Cohen H. 2017. https://www.fertstertdialog.com/users/16110-fertility-and-sterility/posts/19876-klonoff-cohen-consider-this

[148] Dighiero G, Lymberi P, Holmberg D, Lundquist I, Coutinho A, Avrameas S. High frequency of natural autoantibodies mice in normal Newborn. Journal of Immunology. 1985;**134**(2):765-771. PMID: 4038410

[149] Dighiero G, Guilbert B, Fermand JP, Lymberi P, Danon F, Avrameas S. Thirty-six human monoclonal immunoglobulins with antibody activity against cytoskeleton proteins, thyroglobulin, and native DNA: Immunologic studies and clinical correlations. Blood. 1983; **62**(2):264-270. PMID: 6409187

[150] Savitskaya YA, Duarte C, Marín N, Téllez R, Alfaro A, Ibarra C. Identification of circulating natural antibodies against endogenous mediators in the peripheral blood sera of patients with osteoarthritis of the knee: A new diagnostic frontier. Journal of Molecular Biomarkers & Diagnosis. 2012;**3**:135. DOI: 10.4172/2155-9929.1000135

[151] Zhen X, Qiao J, Li R, Wang L, Ping L. Serologic autoimmunologic parameters in women with primary ovarian insufficiency. BMC Immunology. 2014;**15**:11. PMID: 24606591. DOI: 10.1186/1471-2172-15-11

[152] Cline AM, Kutteh WH. Is there a role of autoimmunity in implantation failure after in-vitro fertilization? Current Opinion in Obstetrics & Gynecology. 2009;**21**(3):291-295. PMID: 19469047

[153] Boumpas DT, Chrousos GP, Wilder RL, Cupps TR, Balow JE. Glucocorticoid therapy for immune mediated diseases: Basic and clinical correlates. Annals of Internal Medicine. 1993;**119**:1198-1208. PMID: 8239251

[154] Boumpas DT, Austin HA 3rd, Vaughan EM, Yarboro CH, Klippel JH, Balow JE. Risk for sustained amenorrhea in patients with systemic lupus erythematosus receiving intermittent pulse cyclophosphamide therapy. Annals of Internal Medicine. 1993;**119**(5):366-369. PMID: 8338289

[155] Otsuka N, Tong Z-B, Vanevski K, Tu W, Cheng MH, Nelson LM. Autoimmune oophoritis with multiple molecular targets mitigated by transgenic expression of mater. Endocrinology. 2011;**152**(6):2465-2473. PMID: 21447630. DOI: 10.1210/en.2011-0022

[156] Zhang D, Tu E, Kasagi S, Zanvit P, Chen Q, Chen W. Manipulating regulatory T cells: A promising strategy to treat autoimmunity. Immunotherapy. 2015;**7**:1201, 11. PMID: 26568117-1211. DOI: 10.2217/imt.15.79

[157] Vojdani A. Antibodies as predictors of complex autoimmune diseases. International Journal of Immunopathology and Pharmacology. 2008;**21**:267-278. PMID: 18547471. DOI: 10.1177/039463200802100203

[158] Busnelli A, Paffoni A, Fedele L, Somigliana E. The impact of thyroid autoimmunity on IVF/ICSI outcome: A systematic review and meta-analysis. Human Reproduction Update. 2016;**22**(6):775-790. PMID: 27323769. DOI: 10.1093/humupd/dmw019

[159] Unuane D, Velkeniers B, Anckaert E, Schiettecatte J, Tournaye H, Haentjens P, Poppe K. Thyroglobulin autoantibodies: Is there any added value in the detection of thyroid autoimmunity in women consulting for fertility treatment? Thyroid. 2013;**23**(8):1022-1028. PMID: 23405888. DOI: 10.1089/thy.2012.0562

Section 2

Cytokines and Interferons

Chapter 4

Cytokines and Interferons: Types and Functions

Vinicius L. Ferreira, Helena H.L. Borba,
Aline de F. Bonetti, Leticia P. Leonart and
Roberto Pontarolo

Additional information is available at the end of the chapter

http://dx.doi.org/10.5772/intechopen.74550

Abstract

This chapter aims to describe and review the main important cytokines types (notably interferons), including their biological activities, functions and structures. As a high number of molecules are available, synthesis of the most important cytokines, including tumor factor necrosis, interferons and interleukins will be presented. Here we also describe the relationships between those cytokines with some autoimmune diseases that are promoted by them.

Keywords: biological function, cytokines, interferon, tumor factor necrosis, interleukins

1. Introduction

Cytokines are a cell-signaling group of low molecular weight extracellular polypeptides/glycoproteins synthesized by different immune cells, mainly, by T cells, neutrophils and macrophages, which are responsible to promote and regulate immune response (i.e. activity, differentiation, proliferation and production of cells and other cytokines). These polypeptides act on signaling molecules and cells, stimulating them toward sites of inflammation, infections, traumas, acting on primary lymphocyte growth factors and other biological functions. Cytokines may act in the site where they are produced (autocrine action), in nearby cells (paracrine action) or in distant cells (endocrine action). In this sense, they are important in the development and regulation of immune system cells. Different types of cytokines had been discovered, including chemokines, interferons (IFN), interleukins (IL), lymphokines and tumor necrosis factor (TNF) [1–4].

In this chapter, we describe and review different cytokines. They will be categorized according to their type, followed by presentation of their function and a brief scope: IFN (IFN-α, β and γ), IL (IL-1, IL-2 and others), TNF (TNF-α and TNF-β) and others. A brief explanation of different cytokines activities also will be done, comprising pro- and anti-inflammatory action, cellular immune responses and performance in hematopoiesis. Methods to reach these objectives include a literature search in the most relevant sources of information, including PubMed/Medline, Scopus and Web of Science databases.

As key results, this chapter will provide a better understanding on cytokines types and functions, with organized concepts about this subject. As we aim to provide a comprehensive review of the available data regarding cytokines, this chapter will be a valuable source of information for readers who seek a thorough and structured synthesis on this topic.

2. Interferons

Interferon family represents a widely expressed group of cytokines. It includes three main classes, designated as type I IFNs, type II IFN and type III IFNs. The two main type I IFNs includes IFN-α (further classified into 13 different subtypes such as IFN-α1, -α2, -α4, -α5, -α6, -α7, -α8, -α10, -α13, -α14, -α16, -α17 and -α21), and IFN-β. The term *interferon* derives from the ability of these cytokines to interfere with viral replication. Type I IFNs present a potent antiviral effect by inhibiting viral replication, increasing the lysis potential of natural killer (NK) cells and the expression of MHC class I molecules on virus-infected cells, and stimulating the development of Th1 cells. During an infectious process, this type of interferon becomes abundant and is easily detectable in the blood. On the other hand, type II IFN has only one representative, IFN-γ. This cytokine plays a major role is macrophage activation both in innate and adaptive immune responses. Type III IFNs, also denoted IL-28/29, present similar biological effects to type I IFN, playing an important role in host defense against viral infections [5–8].

2.1. History

Interferon was the first described member of the class of protein molecules now known as cytokines. Nowadays, interferons are well known to participate in innate immune system, mediating responses against viral infections. This role of the IFNs was first described in the 1930s, when a research conducted by Hoskins demonstrated that rabbits previously infected by the herpes simplex virus were protected against subsequent infections by the same type of virus. In 1937, a few years after Hoskins' experiment, Findlay and MacCallum showed that the virus-infected animals were also resistant to infections caused by antigenically different viruses, corroborating and complementing the existing evidence regarding IFNs functions at that time. Their findings, however, were only confirmed in 1957, when Isaacs and Lindenmann, through cell cultures research, demonstrated that cells infected by a virus had the ability to produce a protein that could make other cells resistant to other viruses. Glasgow, in 1966, theorized that the interferon production was not limited to primary infection by viruses, and that this cytokine might play a role following re-infection. Therefore, the concept of "immune induction" of interferon became well established by the end of the 1960s. The early 1970s were marked by two milestone studies, which confirmed the existence of two different categories of interferons, which differed physicochemically and biologically: the immune-induced interferon (currently known as type II IFN) and the classical virus-induced interferon (currently known as type I IFN). In 1980, the terms IFN-α and IFN-β arose to designate the "classical interferons", which had been obtained in pure forms exhibiting homogeneity. Albeit the "immune-induced interferon" had not been obtained in pure form at that time, it was recognized that this molecule was different from IFN-α and IFN-β, being, therefore, designated as IFN-γ. Despite the markedly difference of this cytokine when compared to IFN-α and IFN-β, IFN-γ was originally classified in the IFN family due to its ability to 'interfere' with viral infections, which characterizes the original definition of IFNs. In the last decade, a third type of IFN (type III IFN) has been described, the IFN-λ. This type is also referred as interleukins IL-28A and B (IFN-λ2 and IFN-λ3, respectively), and IL-29 (IFN-λ1) [8–11].

2.2. Pathways of induction and major roles of interferons

There are several isotypes of type I IFNs. In humans, there are multiple forms of IFN-α, only one type of IFN-β and additional isotypes, as IFN-δ, IFN-ε, IFN-κ, IFN-τ and IFN-ω (IFN-δ and IFN-τ have been only described in pigs and cattle). This sort of cytokines presents similar structure, binding to the same cell surface receptor, and they are coded by a family of linked genes located on the human chromosome 9 [7, 12].

Type I IFN synthesis is induced by microbial challenge (i.e., viral and bacterial infections or microbial nucleic acids exposure) when the pattern recognition receptors (PRRs) sense these microorganisms. These receptors can be found in the cytosol or in the endosome. Once a virus infects a cell, the cell activates signals that lead to phosphorylation, dimerization and passage to the nucleus of the interferon response factor 3 (IRF3). Along with IRF3, other transcription factors, such as nuclear factor kappa B (NF-κB) and activator protein 1 (AP-1), activate the transcription of IFN-β gene. After this process, secreted IFN-β binds to the interferon receptor (IFNAR) on the surface of the infected cell, producing an autocrine signaling to mobilize other interferon response factors and alter gene expression patterns to provide interferon response. Besides autocrine signaling, IFN-β also binds to the interferon receptor expressed by neighboring non-virus infected cells, acting in a paracrine manner to promote interferon response in order to help these cells to resist viral infection [5, 13, 14].

Interferon response comprises a series of reactions that alter the expression of a variety of human genes. These reactions are mediated by the binding with type I interferon receptors, which consists of the IFNAR1 and IFNAR2 transmembrane proteins, and two associated cytoplasmic tyrosine kinases, the Janus kinase 1 (Jak1) and tyrosine kinase 2 (TyK2). In addition to IRF3, another transcription factor induced by interferon response is interferon response factor 7 (IRF7), which is responsible to initiate IFN-α transcription without the need of NF-κB and AP-1. The canonical pathway that mediates the biological effects of IFNs corresponds to the Janus kinase/signal transducer and activator of transcription (JAK/STAT) pathway. Both the antiviral and inflammatory effects of IFN-α/IFN-β are specifically mediated by STAT1 and STAT2. This pathway, however, does not work in isolated manner. It extensively communicates with other signal transduction pathways, therefore recruiting several effector molecules to promote a potent effect against viral infections, antiproliferative and antitumor activities, in addition to the immunomodulatory effects. In healthy individuals, these type I IFN genes are strictly regulated, with almost no constitutive IFN-α production [7, 15, 16].

A high number of cells produce IFN-α and IFN-β, including macrophages, fibroblasts, and endothelial cells, specialized leukocytes, called interferon-producing cells (IPCs), or natural interferon-producing cells, secrete up to 1000 times more interferon than the others after microbial challenge. These cells, also known as plasmacytoid dendritic cell (pDCs), are present in the blood, comprising less than 1% of the total peripheral blood mononuclear cells. In terms of morphology, they are similar to plasmocytes, another type of cell responsible for the massive production of this cytokine. IPCs express toll-like receptors (TLRs) 6, 7, 9 and 10, which are critical components of innate immunity, acting as pathogen sensors. Toll-like receptors act on innate immunity cells by detecting conserved patterns of pathogenic microorganisms. These cells, when activated by these receptors, lead to maturation of antigen-presenting cells and production of inflammatory cytokines. Hence, IPCs become responsive to a variety of viral infections through quick secretion of massive amounts of type I IFN. In other words, these cells can produce substantial amounts of type I IFN in response to stimulation with a wide range of DNA and RNA viruses, which signal through TLR9 and TLR7, respectively. During an antiviral immune response, therefore, IPCs are able to promote the function of NK cells, B and T cells, and myeloid dendritic cells through type I IFN. IPCs still differentiate into a unique type of mature dendritic cell, which allows the direct regulation of the function of T cells and links innate and adaptive immune responses. This process occurs at a later stage of viral infection [11, 17–20].

The whole process mentioned above can be summarized through the following explanation. On the first day after stimulation by viral infection (microbial challenge), IPCs produce massive amounts of type I IFN. On the following 2 days, IPCs differentiate into a type of dendritic cell called a plasmacytoid dendritic cell, which maintains the ability to produce interferon. During the infection process, these cells cluster into the T cell areas of the draining lymph nodes. Although there is some similarity between plasmacytoid dendritic cells and myeloid dendritic cells (known as conventional dendritic cells), it is believed that plasmacytoid dendritic cells do not have a substantial involvement in T cell activation in adaptive immunity, which is the main function of conventional dendritic cells. Therefore, in the context of innate immunity, conventional dendritic cells produce relatively small amounts of type I IFN, but produce large amounts of IL-12, a cytokine that interacts with type I IFN to activate the NK cell response to viral infection [7, 11].

IFNs, besides being first line of defense against viral infections, play important roles in immunosurveillance for malignant cells. More specifically, type I interferons present a potent antiviral activity, which is associated with several physiological changes. For ease of understanding, the role of type I interferons, in which IFN-α and IFN-β are the major actors, can be divided in three main functions. Firstly, these cytokines stimulate resistance to viral replication in all cells through cellular genes activation, with the consequent destruction of the viral mRNA and inhibition of the viral proteins translation. Secondly, they promote an increase in

http://dx.doi.org/10.5772/intechopen.74550

ligands to NK cell receptors expression in virus-infected cells. Thirdly, they lead to NK cells to eradicate virus-infected cells [8, 21, 22].

NK cells are lymphocytes of innate immune system, which provide defense against viral infections by secreting cytokines (mainly IFN-γ) and killing infected cells. When IFN-α or IFN-β bind to interferon receptors on circulating NK cells, these are activated and directed to infected tissues, where they attack virus-infected cells. It is possible to say that NK cells play, in innate immune response, similar functions than cytotoxic T cells in adaptive immune response [23, 24].

Type II and type III IFNs do not share homogeneity with type I IFN in terms of induction, and the signaling pathways are, therefore, through their own receptors. Nevertheless, the signal pathways involved with type I IFN and type II IFN, as well as the target genes used by these cytokines, somewhat overlap. IFN-γ receptor (IFNGR) is composed by two structurally homologous polypeptides that belong to the type II cytokine receptor family, named IFN-γR1 and IFN-γR2. IFN-γ (originally designated as macrophage-activating factor) binds and induces dimerization of the two receptor chains. This process leads to the activation of JAK1 and JAK2 kinases and, subsequently, to the phosphorylation and dimerization of STAT1, which stimulates the transcription of several genes. The genes induced by this cytokine encode several different molecules that mediate the biological activities of IFN-γ [5, 14, 25].

Unlike IFN-α or IFN-β, the gene that encodes IFN-γ is located on the human chromosome 12. This unique specimen of type II IFN is the primary cytokine involved in macrophage activation (named as classical activation) and plays a critical role in immunity against intracellular microorganisms. In innate immune system, IFN-γ is the main cytokine produced by NK cells, acting as a mediator of innate immunity. Despite belonging to the *interferon* family, IFN-γ does not produce a potent antiviral effect, running primarily as an activator of effector cells of the immune system. In adaptive immunity, IFN-γ is produced by T cells in response to antigen recognition, and its secretion is increased by IL-12 and IL-18. In addition, B cells and professional antigen-presenting cells (e.g., monocyte/macrophage and dendritic cells) are also involved in this cytokine production. While IL-12 and IL-18 control the production of IFN-γ by promoting its synthesis, IL-4 and IL-10 correspond to the negative regulators of type II IFN production [5, 8, 25].

Regarding biological activities, both type I and type II IFN are essential in the immediate cellular response to viral infections. IFN-γ acts on immune cell activation and induction of the major histocompatibility complex (MHC) molecules, which is important at a later stage of the response. Thus, this cytokine establishes an antiviral state for long-term control, coordinating the transition from innate to adaptive immunity. IFN-γ plays a role in macrophage activation, triggering microbicide effector functions in these cells. Macrophages activated by IFN-γ promote more intensive pinocytosis and phagocytosis, in addition to an improved microbial killing ability. Furthermore, IFN-γ acts as a cell growth inhibitor and presents the ability of triggering apoptosis [25, 26].

In summary, in the early stages of infection, NK cells are the main producers of IFN-γ, whose major role is macrophage activation. Once activated, macrophages release cytokines that participate in T cells activation, therefore initiating the adaptive immune response. After being produced and entering the infected site, the effector T cells become, in turn, the main source of IFN-γ and cell-mediated cytotoxicity. Besides the effects on host defense, IFN-γ is also involved in the protection against tumor development [5, 26].

Type III IFN (IL-28/29 or IFN-λ), likewise type I IFN, present antiviral activity. Type III IFN is subdivided in IFN-λ1 and IFN-λ2/3, which are expressed in identical patterns. The signaling pathway related to IFN-λ is similar to IFN-α/IFN-β, involving mechanisms relying on IRFs and NF-κB actions, with the last one playing an essential role in regulating type III IFN expression. Nevertheless, the expression of IFN-λ is more flexible when compared to type I IFN, once it also involves independent actions of NF-kB and IRFs, allowing the production of this cytokine in response to a wider range of stimuli. Most classes of virus and some bacterial products induce IFN-λ expression, and almost all cell types, mostly pDCs, produce type III IFN after virus infection. However, different from the other types of IFN, macrophages are not involved in IFN-λ expression. Regarding biological activities, IFN-λ acts as the first line in host defense against viral infections, besides regulating innate and adaptive immune responses. Recently, a new member of the Interferon Lambda family was identified, the IFN-λ4. This cytokine presents strong antiviral activity and has been recently described to be related to hepatitis C treatment failure. Several *in vivo* studies have shown that IFN-λ can be developed as a potent antiviral agent, covering a wide spectrum of viral infections, with the additional benefit of not promoting the unwanted pro-inflammatory effects of IFN-α [6, 27–29].

2.3. Interferons and related diseases

The first sign that type I IFN was somehow involved with human autoimmune diseases came from the observation of an increased incidence of autoantibodies and autoimmune diseases after type I IFN treatment. Hence, when considering the indication of IFN-α therapy for some conditions (e.g., hepatitis C virus infection), it is important to scrutinize the presence of autoantibodies in the patient, since they may increase the risk for autoimmune disease development with this kind of treatment [14]. As previously mentioned, pDCs are responsible for producing high levels of type I IFN in response to nucleic acid-containing immune complexes through the activation of TLRs 7 and 9 [11]. These immune complexes are prevalent in autoimmune conditions, such as systemic lupus erythematosus (SLE), which makes this process highly relevant for the development of autoimmunity. It has been described that, in autoimmune diseases, several key immune effector cells, such as B cells, T effector cells and regulatory T cells are modulated by IFN-α. Hence, type I IFN plays a substantial role in this kind of condition [16].

Regarding type II IFN, IFN-γ may contribute to the pathogenesis of autoimmune diseases, such as systemic lupus erythematosus, multiple sclerosis and type I diabetes mellitus. The role of this cytokine in autoimmune diseases (both in promoting and suppressing the condition) has been shown in several mouse models. The administration of IFN-γ at very early stages of experimental autoimmune encephalomyelitis exacerbates the disease, while its administration at a later stage reduces disease severity. Hence, the absence of biomarkers that could indicate the best stage of the disease to initiate IFN-γ treatment consists in a limiting factor for its therapeutic use [25, 26, 30]. This subject will be reported in the topic "Cytokines and autoantibodies".

Due to the ability to increase immune response, type I and type II IFN have been explored in clinical trials as treatments for several conditions. It has been found that these cytokines are involved with the improvement of several conditions, such as hepatitis B and C virus infections, autoimmune diseases and certain types of leukemia and lymphomas. Hence, this class of cytokines, which play a paramount role in the immune system, consist of valuable treatment strategy. Still, in order to obtain full advantage of the therapeutic potential of interferons, further researches are needed to elucidate the core mechanisms of their effects [31, 32].

3. Tumor necrosis factor

Tumor necrosis factor (TNF) is a cytokine that had the name derived from it discovery in 1975 as a molecule that caused in vitro necrosis of tumors. Shortly thereafter, it was observed that TNF expression was promoted by immune system cells. These discoveries were important to a posterior characterizing of the TNF superfamily and the TNF receptor superfamily, which has more than 40 members, being the most outstanding TNF-α (commonly named as TNF) and TNF-β (also named Iymphotoxin), but also including cytokines and membrane proteins that have similar sequence homologies and a homotrimeric pyramidal structure (e.g. CD40 ligand, FAS ligand, OX40 ligand, GITR ligand and other several proteins). The binding of this family of cytokines with their respective receptors triggers especially inflammatory reactions [33–37] .

TNF-β, a type II transmembrane protein, is an important key in the development of lymph nodes and Peyer's patches, and also for the maintenance of secondary lymphoid organs. The expression of TNF-β is mainly stimulated by lymphocytes. TNF-α will be better described in the following topics [38, 39].

Although it were discovered many receptors along the decades, two are best known: TNFR1 (55 kD) and TNFR2 (75 kD). Both receptors are plasma membrane trimmers, while TNFR1 is expressed by most human cells and TNFR2 is mainly produced by immune system cells. It is important to mention that TNFR2 have a higher affinity to TNF. They are related to inflammatory reactions, so that a cytokine bind to the receptor, it induces the recruitment of proteins that are important for the process [35, 40] .

3.1. Expression and structure of tumor necrosis factor alpha

The production of this cytokine is performed by different cells from the immune system, which includes T cells, NK cells, macrophages and monocytes. The stimulus for TNF expression includes different factors, such as bind to pathogen lipopolysaccharide (LPS) and other parts with toll-like receptors (TLRs), and also by other cytokines, highlighting IFN-y [33, 35].

It is primary secreted as a nonglycosylated type II membrane protein arranged as homotrimer. TNF membrane releases a trimeric soluble cytokine (a polypeptide that weighs around 17-kDa with triangular pyramid shape) through proteolytic cleavage by metalloprotease TNF-converting enzyme, and this is the circulating form that is found in blood plasma, and that allows a potent capacity to displacement in the body, thus it endocrine function. It is not well defined but from three of these circulating TNF it is possible to polymerize them forming one 51-kD polypeptide which facilitates the binding of the cytokine with three receptors simultaneously [37, 41, 42].

3.2. Tumor necrosis factor alpha biologic functions

TNF have a lot of physiologic multifunction including immune and inflammatory roles and the survival and death of different cells. The main function of cytokine is to attract and activate immune cells to sites of infections and to destroy pathogens, such as bacteria and virus. In this context, TNF stimulate vascular endothelial cells to express adhesion molecules (e.g. selectins and ligands for leukocyte integrins) that allows immune system cells to connect the wall of blood vessels. Additionally, complementing the inflammatory response, TNF induces the production of chemokines that increase the affinity of leukocyte to their ligands, the expression of IL-1 and to activate microbicidal functions of immune system cells. For all TNF importance in the inflammatory reaction, if low quantities of this cytokine are presented in the local, the containment of the infection may be impaired [33, 37, 41–43].

TNF is also well known to act in inflammatory reaction of some autoimmune diseases, such as rheumatoid arthritis and inflammatory bowel disease. Errors in this production are responsible for a considerable number of autoimmune, neoplastic and other diseases. Under these conditions, the treatment of these diseases are based on biologic agents targeting TNF, and thus looking for reducing the number of available TNF molecules or to block it receptors [33, 35, 40].

TNF also promotes necrosis of tumor cells by inducing programmed cell death, a cytolytic potential. The activation of apoptosis mechanism is mediated by TNFR1, by stimulating the recruitment of death signaling proteins, such as Fas-associated protein with death, TNFR-associated factor (TRAF)-1 and TNFR-associated death domain protein (TRADD). These intracellular proteins are responsible for the release of other proteins such as pro-caspase-8, which in it activated form activate caspase-3, caspase-6, caspase-7 and other cytosolic substrates. These proteins induce genomic DNA degradation and cell death through interacting with latent DNAse. Evidences also suggest that TNF have the capacity to induce carcinogenesis and to stabilize tumors, an event that it is opposite of the previous explained, by DNA mutations and it mechanism of repair (i.e. genotoxic potential). This is possible due to the activation of NF-κB in tumor cells and by promoting production of IL-6 (a tumor-promoting cytokine), both facilitate metastasis and cancer cells to escape from immune system defense [35, 40–42].

There are other biological events and actions caused by TNF. When this cytokine is produced in large scale, such as in severe infection, it may induce shock or decrease of blood pressure due to reducing vascular muscle tone and myocardial contractility. Additionally, in high concentrations TNF can reduce blood glucose concentration, and cause intravascular thrombosis (by decreasing anticoagulant capabilities of the endothelium). TNF is also known as an endogenous pyrogen because it promotes fever by stimulating hypothalamus cells to produce prostaglandins [33, 40].

4. Interleukins

Interleukins (ILs) are a group of secreted proteins with diverse structures and functions. These proteins bind to receptors and are involved in the communication between leukocytes. They are intimately related with activation and suppression of the immune system and cell division. The interleukins are synthesized mostly by helper $CD4^+$ T lymphocytes, monocytes, macrophages and endothelial cells [5, 44, 45].

Interleukins are named as IL plus a number. Previously, different names were used to refer to the same IL. For instance, IL-1 was called lymphocyte-activating factor, mitogenic protein or T cell replacing factor III. In order to standardize the nomenclature, in 1979, during the Second International Lymphokine Workshop, the term interleukin was introduced. After that, the interleukins started being named consecutively according to the date of their discovery [44, 46, 47].

There have been identified 40 interleukins so far and some of them are further divided into subtypes (e.g. IL-1α, IL-1β). These ILs are grouped in families based on sequence homology and receptor chain similarities or functional properties [5, 44, 48, 49].

In this section, a brief description of various ILs will be presented. Focus will be given to the families of interleukins 1 and 2.

4.1. The interleukin-1 family

Interleukin-1 family is composed by 11 cytokines: 7 ligands with agonist activity (IL-1α, IL-1β, IL-18, IL-33, IL-36α, IL-36β and IL-36γ), 3 receptor antagonists (IL-1Ra, IL-36Ra and IL-38) and 1 anti-inflammatory cytokine (IL-37) [44, 50].

The interleukin-1 family started with only two components: IL-1α, IL-1β. Over the years, new IL with similar behavior and/or structure were discovered and added to the family. All the agonists members of this family show pro-inflammatory activity. These cytokines share a common C-terminal three-dimensional structure with a typical β-trefoil fold consisting of 12-β-strands connected by 11 loops, and have identical positioning of certain introns. Considering that, it is plausible to affirm that they probably arose from the duplication of a common ancestral gene [45, 51, 52].

All members of the family except IL-18 and IL-33 have genes encoding on chromosome 2 in a 400 kb region in human species. Despite the fact that all the cytokines are extracellular, they are synthesized without a hydrophobic leader sequence and are not secreted via reticulum endoplasmic-Golgi pathway, with the exception of IL-1Ra. The secretion mechanism of the other members of the family is still not known. These cytokines bind to closely related receptors, and many of the encoding genes are clustered in a short region of chromosome 2. The receptors contain extracellular immunoglobulin domains and a toll/IL-1 receptor (TIR) domain in the cytoplasmic portion [45, 52].

In order to become active, both IL-1α and IL-1β bind to the ligand-binding chain type I (IL-1R1). Then, the co-receptor, termed the accessory protein (IL-1RAcP), is recruited, and together they form a heterodimeric complex. The signaling that will culminate in a variety of inflammatory activities is initiated by the recruitment of the adaptor protein MyD88 to the toll-IL-1 receptor (TIR), which is followed by the phosphorylation of kinases, the translocation of the nuclear factor kappa B (NF-κB) to the nucleus and the expression of inflammatory genes [50, 51].

Both IL-1α and IL-1β have precursor forms. The precursor of IL-1α is present in the epithelial layers of the gastrointestinal tract, lung, liver, kidney, endothelial cells and astrocytes; and it is capable of binding to the IL-1R1 and initiating the signaling cascade, essentially after cell death by necrosis (e.g. myocardial infarction and stroke). On the other hand, the precursor of IL-1β is not active and does not bind to the receptor. It requires a cleavage to become in the active form [44, 50, 51].

IL-1β is highly involved with autoimmune, infectious, degenerative and, especially, with autoinflammatory diseases. An important part of autoinflammatory diseases is caused by genetic defects in innate inflammatory pathways, and usually show their signals early in life. The first disease classified as autoinflammatory was tumor necrosis factor receptor associated periodic syndrome (TRAPS). Other examples are familial Mediterranean fever and adult and juvenile Still disease. This group of diseases promptly responds to the treatment with IL-1β blockade, with few exceptions. In many autoinflammatory diseases, there is a state of increased release of IL-1β. The precursor is converted to the active form through the action of Caspase-1. This enzyme is also found in the inactive form in tissue macrophages and dendritic cells, and requires conversion by autocatalysis to become active. However, it is in the active form in circulating human blood monocytes. The release of IL-1β from blood monocytes in highly controlled and takes several hours in healthy subjects. In patients with an autoinflammatory disease, more mature IL-1β is released when compared to healthy subjects, which leads to exacerbated inflammation. Despite of this group of diseases being characterized by severe inflammation, the amount of IL-1β released is not much greater than that released from healthy subjects. Currently, human anti-IL-1β monoclonal antibody is being developed to treat autoinflammatory diseases. Canakinumab was approved by Food and Drug Administration (FDA) in 2009 for the treatment of cryopyrin-associated periodic syndromes (CAPS). In 2016, Canakinumab was also approved for treating TRAPS, hyperimmunoglobulin D syndrome (HIDS)/mevalonate kinase deficiency (MKD) and familial Mediterranean fever (FMF) [50, 51].

IL-1Ra is a receptor antagonist. It is synthetized by the same cells that produce IL-1α and IL-1β (monocytes, macrophages, dendritic cells and others). The binding of IL-1Ra to the receptor does not involve conformational change and, hence, the co-receptor IL-1RAcP is not recruited. IL-1Ra regulates the activity of IL-1. However, to efficiently block the IL-1 response, it has to be in an amount approximately 100-folds greater than the agonists cytokines. Anakinra is a recombinant version of IL1-Ra used in the treatment of rheumatoid arthritis [44, 53].

IL-18 is synthetized as an inactive precursor, and, similarly to IL-1β, it needs cleavage by caspase-1 to become in the active form. The precursor form is present in almost all cells of the human body, likewise IL-1α. Usually diseases related to IL-18 appear when there is an imbalance between the amount of IL-18 and IL-18 binding protein, which is responsible for limiting the level of activity of IL-18. This cytokine is released usually from dying cells, once again like IL-1α [51, 54].

IL-18 was first described as "IFN-γ-inducing factor", because it was discovered as an inducer of IFN-γ production. However, alone, IL-18 does not induce the production of considerable amounts of IFN-γ. For that to happen, it has to act in association with IL-12. IL-18 promotes TH_1 and Th_2 cells responses, and also induces IL-13 production in T cells and NK cells together with IL-2. It also enhances NK toxicity by promoting the expression of Fas ligand in NK cells. IL-18 is involved in several autoimmune diseases, in myocardial infarction, metabolic syndromes and others [44, 55].

IL-33 is an alarmin cytokine, rapidly released upon cellular damage. It is involved mainly in type 2 immunity and inflammation. It acts in Th_2, in innate lymphoid cell-2 (ILC2), and in activated M2 polarized macrophages. This cytokine is expressed by keratinocytes, epithelial and endothelial cells, and monocytes. IL-33 is produced as a precursor, but, contrary to IL-1, caspase-1 transforms it in an inactive cytokine. The precursor is active and other proteases can cleavage it in more potent forms. IL-33 induces Th_2 response binding to ST2 and next recruiting IL-1RacP. The activity of IL-33 is controlled essentially by the binding to soluble ST2 and soluble IL-1RAcP. Levels of increased soluble ST2 are present in various inflammatory diseases, such as systemic lupus erythematosus and rheumatoid arthritis [44, 50, 56].

IL-36α, IL-36β and IL-36γ are receptor agonists, while IL-36Ra is a receptor antagonist that blocks the activation of the receptor and competes with IL-36, acting as a regulator. These cytokines are included in the interleukin-1 family because they share homology to the first members of the family. Their homology to IL-Ra and IL-1β varies from 20 to 52%. Furthermore, IL-36β and IL-36γ have the core 12-fold, β-trefoil structure and lack a signal peptide, particular features of IL-1 family. All these cytokines need an N-terminal processing to become in the active form, but the enzyme responsible for this process is still not known. IL-36 cytokines are predominantly found in skin cells, and that is why they are related with several skin disorders, such as psoriasis. After binding to the receptor (IL-36R and IL-1RAcP co-receptor), dendritic cells are activated and participate in the polarizing of T-helper responses [50, 52, 57].

Different from the other members of the family, IL-37 is an anti-inflammatory cytokine, and reduces innate inflammation as well as acquired immune responses. Its presence has already been reported in skin, tonsils, esophagus, placenta, breast, prostate and colon. There are five different isoforms of IL-37: IL-37a, IL-37b, IL-37c, IL-37d and IL-37e, expressed in different locations of the human body. So far, IL-37b, which contains a 12β-strand trefoil, typical of the IL-1 family, appears to be the most biologically active, and therefore the object of the majority of studies. IL-37 suppresses the production of pro-inflammatory cytokines, such as IL-1A, IL-6, CC chemokine ligand (CCL-12), colony-stimulating factors (CSF-1 and CSF-2), chemokine ligand-13 (CXCL-13), IL-1β, IL23-A and IL1RA, and also inhibits dendritic cell activation [58–60].

IL-38 is the most recent member of the Interleukin-1 family, identified in 2001. It binds to the same receptor that the IL-36 cytokines, IL-36R. However, it acts as an antagonist, similarly to IL-36Ra. Therefore, IL-38 acts reducing inflammatory response. IL-38 shares 41% homology with IL-1Ra and 43% with IL-36Ra. This cytokine is present in skin, tonsil, thymus, spleen, fetal liver and salivary glands. The properties and biological activities of IL-38 are still being studied [52, 61, 62].

4.2. Interleukin-2 family

The IL-2 cytokine family, also known as the common γ-chain family, is composed by ILs 2, 4, 7, 9, 15 and 21. All these ILs bind to the common γc receptor, also called CD132. These cytokines act as growth and proliferation factors for progenitors and mature cells [44, 63].

IL-2 is the first member of the common γ-chain family, previously known as T cell growth factor. This cytokine is mainly produced by $CD4^+$ and $CD8^+$ T cells, but can be also expressed by dendritic cells and NKs. The IL-2R is composed by three subunits (CD25, CD122 and common γc), all necessary to binding to IL-2. IL-2 acts in the development of regulatory T (Treg) cells, as a B cell growth factor, stimulates antibody synthesis and promotes proliferation and differentiation of NK cells and T helpers. IL-2 has been extensively used as an anti-cancer therapy [44, 63–65].

IL-4 is produced by Th_2 cells, basophils, eosinophils and mastocytes. It has two receptors: IL4-R type I, which binds only to IL-4 and is composed by CD124 (IL-4rα) and CD 132; and type II, which binds to IL-4 and to IL-13, and it consists in IL-4Rα and IL-13Rα1. These receptors are spread all over the human body. IL-4 is known to play several different roles, regulating allergic conditions and activating the immune response against extracellular parasites (B cell class switching to IgE). It is the main cytokine to stimulate development of Th_2 cells. Dupilimab is an IL-4 receptor antagonist approved in 2017 by FDA for treatment of eczema [44, 66, 67].

IL-7 is a homeostatic cytokine. It can be found essentially in T cells, progenitors of B cells and bone marrow macrophages. As the other members of the family, its receptor (IL-7R) consists in the common γ-chain fraction, along with another unit, the IL-7Rα (CD127). IL-7 is involved in the survival and proliferation of thymocytes and in the development of naïve and memory B and T cells, mature T cells and NKs. Deficiencies related to IL-7 result in immunodeficiency, autoimmune diseases and leukemia [44, 68].

IL-9 is mainly produced by Th_2 cells, but it is also expressed in less amounts by eosinophils and by mastocytes of asthmatic patients. Its receptor, IL-9R, is composed by the CD132 and IL-9Rα units. IL-9 is a potent growth factor for T cells and mastocytes, and some of it activities include the inhibition of cytokine production by Th_1 cells, IgE production, and mucus secretion by bronchial epithelium. Recently, a new subset of effector T cells was discovered, Th_9, and it is believed that it is intimately related with IL-9 production. IL-9 is associated to allergic diseases and protection from helminthic infections. This cytokine can be found in elevated amounts in Hodgkin lymphoma, hence, IL-9 antagonists are being studied as a potential treatment for this disease [44, 69, 70].

IL-15 is structurally homologous to IL-2. The receptor, IL-15R, is composed by the CD132 subunit common to the family, and also by IL-15Rα and IL-2Rβ chains. IL-15 is produced by keratinocytes, skeletal muscle cells, monocytes and activated $CD4^+$ T cells, in response to signals that trigger innate immunity. IL-15 has some identical functions to IL-2, such as T cell activation and stimulation of NK cell proliferation, but it also involved with $CD8^+$ memory cell, NK cell, and NKT-cell homeostasis. Increased levels of IL-15 were reported in autoimmune disorders, such as rheumatoid arthritis, psoriasis and celiac disease [44, 71].

IL-21 is produced by T cells, NKT cells and Th_{17}. The receptor, IL-21, is present in various parts of the human body and consists in CD132 and IL-21R. This cytokine is involved with B cells functions, and also increases the proliferation of $CD8^+$ T cells, NK cells and NKT. IL-21 is currently being studied as anti-cancer therapy [44, 64].

5. Other cytokines

In addition to the aforementioned cytokines, other also deserves attention, such as chemokines. The chemokines represent a large family of structurally homologous cytokines that stimulate leukocytes movement and regulate the migration of them from the blood to tissues, in a process named chemotaxis. They control homeostatic immune cells, such as neutrophils, B cells, and monocytes, trafficking between the bone marrow, blood and peripheral tissues. Therefore, they can be classified as chemotactic cytokines [33, 72].

There are about 50 human chemokines, classified into 4 families according to the location of N-terminal cysteine residues. The two major families are CC and CXC chemokines, in which the cysteine residues are adjacent on CC family, and are separated by one amino acid on CXC family. In general, members of CC chemokines are chemotactic for monocytes, and a small subset of lymphocytes, while CXC chemokines are more specific for neutrophils. The best-known chemokine is IL-8, or CXCL8, which belongs to the CXC chemokine family, and is responsible for neutrophil recruitment and for the maintenance of the inflammatory reaction. On the other hand, the monocyte chemoattractant protein-1 (MCP-1) or CCL2, and CCL11 or eotaxin, are examples of CC chemokines, which acts on recruitment of a variety of leukocytes, but especially monocytes, and eosinophils, respectively [33, 73, 74].

The chemokines receptors are expressed on all leukocytes and are divided in two groups: G protein-coupled receptors with seven-transmembrane α-helical segments, and atypical receptors, which appear to attenuate inflammation by scavenging chemokines, independently of G protein. Each receptor subtype is capable of binding to various chemokines of the same family, and a single chemokine can bind to more than one receptor. Despite of this factor, a lot of chemokines presents a great tissue and receptor specificity [72, 73].

Chemokines can be produced constitutively in various tissues, and are responsible for regulating the traffic of leucocytes, especially lymphocytes, through peripheral lymphoid tissues. However, the best-known activity of chemokines is the involvement on inflammatory reactions. Recruitment of macrophages, neutrophils and T cells to the site of inflammation is strongly stimulated by chemokines. In fact, they represent a secondary pro-inflammatory mediator that is induced by primary pro-inflammatory mediators, such as IL-1 or TNF. In general, members of the chemokines family induce recruitment of well-defined leukocyte subsets, differently of the classic leukocyte chemoattractants. They induce the movement of leukocytes, and consequently promote their migration to a specific local, by stimulating actin filaments [33, 72–74].

Beyond the involvement of the chemokines on acute inflammatory reactions, and the regulation of the traffic of leukocytes through peripheral lymphoid, independently of the presence of inflammation, some kind of chemokines can promote angiogenesis and wound healing, associated mostly with CXC family, while other are involved in the development of diverse nonlymphoid organs [73, 74]. They also have an important role in the priming of naive T cells, in effector and memory cell differentiation, and in regulatory T cell function [72].

Besides chemokines, there are cytokines that stimulates hematopoiesis, such as the colony-stimulating factors (CSFs), which contributes to the growth of progenitors of monocytes, neutrophils, eosinophils and basophils, as well as activating macrophages. Immune and inflammatory reactions uses leukocytes, due to the recruitment induced by some kinds of cytokines, so new must be produced [73, 74]. Additionally, the GM-CSF (granulocyte-macrophage colony-stimulating factor) and M-CSF (macrophage colony-stimulating factor) have, like some other cytokines, a pro-inflammatory action, and exhibit a connexon between the expression of them and TNF, IL-1, IL-23 and IL-17 [75].

Finally, other cytokines can be highlighted: TGF-β, LIF, Eta-1 and oncostatin M. The TGF-β is responsible for the chemoattraction of monocytes and macrophages, but also it has an anti-inflammatory effect, by inhibiting the lymphocyte proliferation. LIF and oncostatin M induce the production of acute-phase protein, while Eta-1 stimulates the production of IL-2, and inhibits the production of IL-10 [73].

6. Cytokines and autoantibodies

On this topic, the association between the cytokines and autoimmune diseases will be reviewed, but emphasis will be given to these ones: systemic lupus erythematosus, type 1 diabetes mellitus, multiple sclerosis, vitiligo and heart failure.

The impossibility of differentiating between own and non-own (strange) could result in the synthesis of antibodies against the components of the organism (autoantibodies), which could be extremely deleterious [73]. The organism is characterized by a failure of the normal mechanism of self-tolerance, resulting in reactions against one's cells, in the absence of any present infection or another cause, known as autoimmunity, and the diseases caused by this phenomenon are referred as autoimmune diseases [33, 76].

The pathogenesis of autoimmune diseases involves mainly the genetic susceptibility, and previous infections. In relation to infections, it is observed a recruitment of leukocytes into the affected tissue, resulting in the activation of tissue antigen-presenting cells (APC). Consequently, these APCs express costimulators and secrete T cell-activating cytokines, contributing to the breakdown of T cell tolerance. Therefore, the infection promotes the activation of T cells that are not specific for the pathogen, in a process called bystander activation. Additionally, microbes may engage toll-like receptors (TRLs) on dendritic cells, resulting on production of lymphocyte-activating cytokines, leading to the autoantibody production. This process was demonstrated in mouse models, and its influence in human autoimmune diseases remains unclear [33].

The systemic lupus erythematosus (SLE) is an autoimmune disease, characterized by the involvement of immune complexes formed from autoantibodies and their specific antigens that are responsible for the clinical manifestation, especially glomerulonephritis, arthritis and vasculitis. The peripheral blood lymphocytes of patient presents an excessive production and response to type 1 IFNs, but the involvement of this cytokines on the development of the diseases is still uncertain [33]. In these patients, for instance, serum IFN-α and IFN-α-induced gene expression are frequently observed, implying that the molecular pathogenesis of this condition is mediated by type I IFN. It has also been shown that IFN-γ serum levels are increased in SLE patients, and in mouse models, the receptor of this cytokine was necessary to the disease development. The massive amount of circulating IFN correlates to disease severity, which is likely to be triggered by excessive pDC activation. Recently, clinical trials evaluating anti-IFN-α monoclonal antibodies for SLE have been conducted, exhibiting promising results. Moreover, a trial evaluating a monoclonal antibody that binds IFN-γ was conducted, but no significant improvements in the efficacy outcome measures were observed. Additionally, a recent study demonstrated that keratinocytes may participate on the pathophysiological of the cutaneous manifestation of the SLE, by increasing cell apoptosis and producing pro-inflammatory cytokines, especially IL-23, IL-12, IL-6, IL-17, (Th17-related cytokines), IL-10 and TFG-β [16, 30, 77, 78].

In parallel, another autoimmune disease widely studied that involves cytokines, besides several other factors, is the type 1 diabetes mellitus. This disease is characterized by pancreatic β cells destruction, which it is due to hypersensitivity reactions mediated by $CD4^+$ TH 1 cells reactive with islet antigens, the effect of cytotoxic T lymphocyte on lysis of islet cells, and local production of cytokines, especially TNF, IL-1, IL-21 and IFN-α. In some cases, the islets show cellular necrosis and lymphocytic infiltration, consisted of both $CD4^+$ and $CD8^+$ cells. Remaining islet cells often express class II MHC molecules, an effect of local production of INF-γ by the T cells [33, 73, 79]. The onset of young age of this disease may be associated with upregulation of growth factors, especially GM-CSF and IL-7. Other mediators overexpressed are the pro-inflammatory cytokine IL-1β, the regulatory cytokine IL-10, IL-27, and some Th17 cytokines (IL-17, IL-21, IL- 23). Additionally, patients that involve to ketoacidosis, a serious complication of the disease, have a tendency for higher IL-8 and IL-10 levels [80].

In the same way, it stands out the rheumatoid arthritis, a chronic and systemic autoimmune disease described as a progressive disability on joints, particularly of the fingers, shoulders, elbows, knees and ankles that can promote systemic consequences like cardiovascular, pulmonary and skeletal disorders. It is characterized by the production of autoantibodies, like rheumatoid factor, cytokines, chemokines, hyperplasic synovium, osteoclastogensis and angiogenesis. The pro-inflammatory cytokines IL-1α/β, IL-8, IL-6, TNF-α, INF-y and some CSFs are responsible for the pathogenesis of this disease, and are involved with the intracellular molecular signaling pathway that causes chronic inflammation on synovial membrane. These cytokines, especially TNF-α, activates the leukocytes endothelial cells and synovial fibroblasts, and stimulates the production of collagenases that are responsible for the destruction of the cartilage, ligaments and tendons of the joints. Therefore, monoclonal antibody drugs, such as anti-TNF are approved for treatment of this disease [33, 75, 76, 81].

It is also believed that bone destruction in rheumatoid arthritis is due to overexpression of the TNF family cytokine receptor activator of nuclear factor KB (RANK), an essential mediator that promotes maturation and activation of osteoclasts [33, 76]. Therefore, the cytokines on rheumatoid arthritis promote the autoimmunity, the destruction of joint tissue and maintain the synovial inflammation [82].

The multiple sclerosis is a neurodegenerative autoimmune disease of high mortality in adults, characterized by a chronic inflammation in the central nervous system with secondary demyelination due to leukocyte and cytokines infiltration of brain tissue and spinal cord. Clinical manifestations are weakness, paralysis and ocular symptoms [33, 73]. A recent study proposed the role of Th1 lymphocytes in the pathogenesis of the brain inflammation, with several cytokines involvement. Th1 lymphocytes produces mainly IFNγ (type II IFN) that is responsible for the production of other pro-inflammatory cytokines, and chemoattractants, such as IL-2, IFNγ, CC chemokines, like CCL5, CCL11 and CCL27 and CXC chemokines, especially CXCL1 and CXCL10. On the other hand, lower levels of circulating type I IFN are observed. Therefore, unlike SLE, multiple sclerosis treatment involves the administration of IFN-β. Additionally, an upregulation of CCL27 was found in cerebrospinal fluid of multiple sclerosis patients, demonstrating the possibility of its involvement on activation and migration of autoreactive immune effectors in the brain, and consequently a potential contribution for the pathogenesis of this disease [83].

Vitiligo, is another autoimmune disease, characterized by the skin depigmentation, which is associated to the production of antibodies against the melanocytes, and it is more frequent in patients that have other autoimmune diseases, like Grave's disease [73]. A variety of cytokines are increased in vitiligo patients in relation to healthy people. A recent systematic review demonstrated an association between the expression of some kind of cytokines in vitiligo skin, especially INF-y, TGF-β, IL-1β, IL-17, and the chemokines CXCL9, CXCL10 and CXCL12. IFN-y and IL-1β are closely related to the pathogenesis of vitiligo, but serum TGF-β and IL-17 are more abundantly expressed in relation to the others [84].

Finally, another disease that has the participation of cytokines on its pathogenesis is the heart failure, a chronic disease characterized by a cardiac impairment due to hypertension, myocardial infarction, arrhythmias and other heart diseases. A recent evidence showed the involvement of the adaptive immune system in the development and progression of heart failure, which is related to high mortality in adults. T cells, particularly TH1, and TH17 and B1 lymphocyte, contribute to the pathologic chronic inflammation, and cell migration. The inflammatory component of this disease, which has a closely relation to the morbidity and mortality, are the cytokines, including TNF-α, TNF-β, IL-1, IL-6, IL-7, IL-10 and IFN-y, chemokines and cardiac autoantibodies. Those factors are associated with cardiomyocyte death and tissue remodeling by fibrosis, contributing to the left ventricle dysfunction, and consequently to disease progression. In detail, initially the dendritic cells and other antigen-presenting cells can process specific proteins of the myocardial tissue and theirs contact with memory B cells promotes the release of autoantibodies, and consequently activates pro-apoptotic pathways, by antigen-dependent cell cytotoxicity, and complement-mediated cell cytotoxicity in health myocytes. Another characteristic of the pathogenesis of heart disease is the production of inflammatory mediators by B cells, such pro-inflammatory cytokines (TNF-α and IL-6) and chemokines, which recruit monocytes involved with inflammation and heart remodeling, beyond the activation of T lymphocytes, leading to the production of other specific inflammatory cytokines (IFN-y and IL-2) [73, 85].

Selective immunosuppression of B-lymphocytes may be a promising therapeutic on acute and chronic heart failure, as the blockage of the immune mediators, such cytokines, once they are involved to the propagation of the disease [85].

In sum, different kinds of cytokines are involved on autoimmune diseases, which plays an important role especially on inflammatory process, and contributing to the pathogenesis, in most cases. Studies have been performed, in order to establish the association between cytokines and the evaluation of these diseases, with the objective of developing therapeutic strategies, such as anti-TNF for rheumatoid arthritis.

7. Conclusion

In this chapter, the main aspects regarding the different types of cytokines and their main functions were reviewed. Hence, the comprehensive and fundamental role of cytokines in the immune system could be thoroughly investigated. Additionally, the contribution of these molecules to the development of diseases, particularly related to autoimmunity, as well as its use as treatment approach for some clinical conditions was explored.

Author details

Vinicius L. Ferreira, Helena H.L. Borba, Aline de F. Bonetti, Leticia P. Leonart and Roberto Pontarolo*

*Address all correspondence to: pontarolo@ufpr.br

Pharmaceutical Sciences Graduate Program, Universidade Federal do Paraná, Curitiba, Paraná, Brazil

References

[1] Zhang JM, An J. Cytokines, inflammation, and pain. International Anesthesiology Clinics. 2007;**45**:27-37

[2] Dinarello CA. Historical review of cytokines. European Journal of Immunology 2007;**37**:S34-S45

[3] Turner MD, Nedjai B, Hurst T, Pennington DJ. Cytokines and chemokines: At the crossroads of cell signalling and inflammatory disease. Biochimica et Biophysica Acta (BBA) – Molecular Cell Research. 2014;**1843**:2563-2582

[4] O'Shea JJ, Ma A, Lipsky P. Cytokines and autoimmunity. Nature Reviews Immunology. 2002;**2**:37-45

[5] Abbas AK, Lichtman AH, Pillai S. Cellular and Molecular Immunology. 8th ed. Philadelphia: Elsevier Saunders; 2015. 535 p

[6] Ank N, West H, Bartholdy C, Eriksson K, Thomsen AR, Paludan SR. Lambda interferon (IFN-lambda), a type III IFN, is induced by viruses and IFNs and displays potent antiviral activity against select virus infections in vivo. Journal of Virology. 2006;**80**:4501-4509

[7] Parham P, Janeway C. The Immune System. 3rd ed. London, New York: Garland Science; 2009. 506 p

[8] Platanias LC. Mechanisms of type-I- and type-II-interferon-mediated signalling. Nature Reviews Immunology. 2005;**5**:375-386

[9] Billiau A, Matthys P. Interferon-gamma: A historical perspective. Cytokine & Growth Factor Reviews. 2009;**20**:97-113

[10] De Andrea M, Ravera R, Gioia D, Gariglio M, Landolfo S. The interferon system: An overview. European journal of paediatric neurology. EJPN: Official Journal of the European Paediatric Neurology Society. 2002;**6**(Suppl A):A41-A46 (discussion A55-8)

[11] Fitzgerald-Bocarsly P, Feng D. The role of type I interferon production by dendritic cells in host defense. Biochimie. 2007;**89**:843-855

[12] Kopitar-Jerala N. The role of interferons in inflammation and Inflammasome activation. Frontiers in Immunology. 2017;**8**:873

[13] Haller O, Kochs G, Weber F. The interferon response circuit: Induction and suppression by pathogenic viruses. Virology. 2006;**344**:119-130

[14] Ronnblom L. The importance of the type I interferon system in autoimmunity. Clinical and Experimental Rheumatology. 2016;**34**:21-24

[15] Ivashkiv LB, Donlin LT. Regulation of type I interferon responses. Nature Reviews Immunology. 2014;**14**:36-49

[16] Lopez de Padilla CM, Niewold TB. The type I interferons: Basic concepts and clinical relevance in immune-mediated inflammatory diseases. Gene. 2016;**576**:14-21

[17] Connolly DJ, O'Neill LA. New developments in toll-like receptor targeted therapeutics. Current Opinion in Pharmacology. 2012;**12**:510-518

[18] Liu YJ. IPC: Professional type 1 interferon-producing cells and plasmacytoid dendritic cell precursors. Annual Review of Immunology. 2005;**23**:275-306

[19] Reynolds JM, Martinez GJ, Chung Y, Dong C. Toll-like receptor 4 signaling in T cells promotes autoimmune inflammation. Proceedings of the National Academy of Sciences of the United States of America. 2012;**109**:13064-13069

[20] Siegal FP, Kadowaki N, Shodell M, Fitzgerald-Bocarsly PA, Shah K, Ho S, et al. The nature of the principal type 1 interferon-producing cells in human blood. Science. 1999;**284**:1835-1837

[21] Gonzalez-Navajas JM, Lee J, David M, Raz E. Immunomodulatory functions of type I interferons. Nature Reviews Immunology. 2012;**12**:125-135

[22] Stackaruk ML, Lee AJ, Ashkar AA. Type I interferon regulation of natural killer cell function in primary and secondary infections. Expert Review of Vaccines. 2013;**12**:875-884

[23] Mandal A, Viswanathan C. Natural killer cells: In health and disease. Hematology/Oncology and Stem Cell Therapy. 2015;**8**:47-55

[24] Vivier E, Tomasello E, Baratin M, Walzer T, Ugolini S. Functions of natural killer cells. Nature Immunology. 2008;**9**:503-510

[25] Schroder K, Hertzog PJ, Ravasi T, Hume DA. Interferon-gamma: An overview of signals, mechanisms and functions. Journal of Leukocyte Biology. 2004;**75**:163-189

[26] Green DS, Young HA, Valencia JC. Current prospects of type II interferon gamma signaling and autoimmunity. The Journal of Biological Chemistry. 2017;**292**:13925-13933

[27] Iversen MB, Paludan SR. Mechanisms of type III interferon expression. Journal of Interferon & Cytokine Research: The Official Journal of the International Society for Interferon and Cytokine Research. 2010;**30**:573-578

[28] Kotenko SV, Durbin JE. Contribution of type III interferons to antiviral immunity: Location, location, location. The Journal of Biological Chemistry. 2017;**292**:7295-7303

[29] O'Brien TR, Prokunina-Olsson L, Donnelly RP. IFN-lambda4: The paradoxical new member of the interferon lambda family. Journal of Interferon & Cytokine Research: The Official Journal of the International Society for Interferon and Cytokine Research. 2014;**34**:829-838

[30] Miller CH, Maher SG, Young HA. Clinical use of interferon-gamma. Annals of the New York Academy of Sciences. 2009;**1182**:69-79

[31] Baker KF, Isaacs JD. Novel therapies for immune-mediated inflammatory diseases: What can we learn from their use in rheumatoid arthritis, spondyloarthritis, systemic lupus erythematosus, psoriasis, Crohn's disease and ulcerative colitis? Annals of the Rheumatic Diseases. 2018;**77**:175-187

[32] Fensterl V, Sen GC. Interferons and viral infections. BioFactors. 2009;**35**:14-20

[33] Abbas AK, Lichtman AH, Pillai S. Cellular and Molecular Immunology. 6th ed. Philadelphia: Saunders Elservier; 2007. 566 p

[34] Abbas AK, Lichtman AH, Pillai SHIV. Imunologia Celular e Molecular. 7th ed. Rio de Janeiro: Elservier; 2012

[35] Brenner D, Blaser H, Mak TW. Regulation of tumour necrosis factor signalling: Live or let die. Nature reviews Immunology. 2015;**15**:362-374

[36] Scheringa M, Marquet RLTNF. A brief review with emphasis on its antitumor activity. Biotherapy (Dordrecht, Netherlands). 1990;**2**:275-281

[37] Ma K, Zhang H, Baloch Z. Pathogenetic and therapeutic applications of tumor necrosis factor-alpha (TNF-alpha) in major depressive disorder: A systematic review. International Journal of Molecular Sciences. 2016;**17**:733

[38] Drutskaya MS, Efimov GA, Kruglov AA, Kuprash DV, Nedospasov SA. Tumor necrosis factor, lymphotoxin and cancer. IUBMB Life. 2010;**62**:283-289

[39] Kuprash DV, Alimzhanov MB, Tumanov AV, Grivennikov SI, Shakhov AN, Drutskaya LN, et al. Redundancy in tumor necrosis factor (TNF) and lymphotoxin (LT) signaling in vivo: Mice with inactivation of the entire TNF/LT locus versus single-knockout mice. Molecular and cellular biology. 2002;**22**:8626-8634

[40] Kalliolias GD, Ivashkiv LB. TNF biology, pathogenic mechanisms and emerging therapeutic strategies. Nature Reviews Rheumatology. 2016;**12**:49-62

[41] Guadagni F, Ferroni P, Palmirotta R, Portarena I, Formica V, Roselli M. Review TNF/VEGF cross-talk in chronic inflammation-related cancer initiation and progression: An early target in anticancer therapeutic strategy. In Vivo (Athens, Greece). 2007;**21**:147-161

[42] Sedger LM, McDermott MF. TNF and TNF-receptors: From mediators of cell death and inflammation to therapeutic giants – Past, present and future. Cytokine & Growth Factor Reviews. 2014;**25**:453-472

[43] Leung L, Cahill CM. TNF-alpha and neuropathic pain – A review. Journal of Neuroinflammation. 2010;**7**:27

[44] Akdis M, Burgler S, Crameri R, Eiwegger T, Fujita H, Gomez E, et al. Interleukins, from 1 to 37, and interferon-gamma: Receptors, functions, and roles in diseases. Journal of Allergy and Clinical Immunology. 2011;**127**:701-721 (e1-70)

[45] Sims JE, Smith DE. The IL-1 family: Regulators of immunity. Nature Reviews Immunology. 2010;**10**:89-102

[46] di Giovine FS, Duff GW. Interleukin 1: The first interleukin. Immunology Today 1990;**11**:13-20

[47] Mizel SB, Farrar JJ. Revised nomenclature for antigen-nonspecific T-cell proliferation and helper factors. Cellular Immunology. 1979;**48**:433-436

[48] Catalan-Dibene J, Vazquez MI, Luu VP, Nuccio SP, Karimzadeh A, Kastenschmidt JM, et al. Identification of IL-40, a novel B cell-associated cytokine. Journal of Immunology. 2017;**199**:3326-3335

[49] Wang X, Wei Y, Xiao H, Liu X, Zhang Y, Han G, et al. A novel IL-23p19/Ebi3 (IL-39) cytokine mediates inflammation in lupus-like mice. European Journal of Immunology. 2016;**46**:1343-1350

[50] Garlanda C, Dinarello CA, Mantovani A. The interleukin-1 family: Back to the future. Immunity. 2013;**39**:1003-1018

[51] Dinarello CA. Interleukin-1 in the pathogenesis and treatment of inflammatory diseases. Blood. 2011;**117**:3720-3732

[52] Palomo J, Dietrich D, Martin P, Palmer G, Gabay C. The interleukin (IL)-1 cytokine family – Balance between agonists and antagonists in inflammatory diseases. Cytokine. 2015;**76**:25-37

[53] Mertens M, Singh JA. Anakinra for rheumatoid arthritis: A systematic review. The Journal of Rheumatology. 2009;**36**:1118-1125

[54] Novick D, Kim S, Kaplanski G, Dinarello CA. Interleukin-18, more than a Th1 cytokine. Seminars in Immunology. 2013;**25**:439-448

[55] Dinarello CA, Novick D, Kim S, Kaplanski G. Interleukin-18 and IL-18 binding protein. Frontiers in Immunology. 2013;**4**:289

[56] Theoharides TC, Petra AI, Taracanova A, Panagiotidou S, Conti P. Targeting IL-33 in autoimmunity and inflammation. The Journal of Pharmacology and Experimental Therapeutics. 2015;**354**:24-31

[57] Gresnigt MS, van de Veerdonk FL. Biology of IL-36 cytokines and their role in disease. Seminars in Immunology. 2013;**25**:458-465

[58] Kumar S, Hanning CR, Brigham-Burke MR, Rieman DJ, Lehr R, Khandekar S, et al. Interleukin-1F7B (IL-1H4/IL-1F7) is processed by caspase-1 and mature IL-1F7B binds to the IL-18 receptor but does not induce IFN-gamma production. Cytokine. 2002;**18**:61-71

[59] Quirk S, Agrawal DK. Immunobiology of IL-37: Mechanism of action and clinical perspectives. Expert Review of Clinical Immunology. 2014;**10**:1703-1709

[60] Xu WD, Zhao Y, Liu Y. Insights into IL-37, the role in autoimmune diseases. Autoimmunity Reviews. 2015;**14**:1170-1175

[61] Kumar S, McDonnell PC, Lehr R, Tierney L, Tzimas MN, Griswold DE, et al. Identification and initial characterization of four novel members of the interleukin-1 family. The Journal of Biological Chemistry. 2000;**275**:10308-10314

[62] Lin H, Ho AS, Haley-Vicente D, Zhang J, Bernal-Fussell J, Pace AM, et al. Cloning and characterization of IL-1HY2, a novel interleukin-1 family member. The Journal of Biological Chemistry. 2001;**276**:20597-20602

[63] Sim GC, Radvanyi L. The IL-2 cytokine family in cancer immunotherapy. Cytokine & Growth Factor Reviews. 2014;**25**:377-390

[64] Lin JX, Leonard WJ. The common cytokine receptor gamma chain family of cytokines. Cold Spring Harbor Perspectives in Biology. 2017 [Epub ahead of print]

[65] Morgan DA, Ruscetti FW, Gallo R. Selective in vitro growth of T lymphocytes from normal human bone marrows. Science. 1976;**193**:1007-1008

[66] Paul WE. History of interleukin-4. Cytokine. 2015;**75**:3-7

[67] Shirley M. Dupilumab: First global approval. Drugs. 2017;**77**:1115-1121

[68] Lundstrom W, Fewkes NM, Mackall CL. IL-7 in human health and disease. Seminars in Immunology. 2012;**24**:218-224

[69] Kaplan MH. Th9 cells: Differentiation and disease. Immunological Reviews. 2013;**252**: 104-115

[70] Zhao P, Xiao X, Ghobrial RM, Li XC. IL-9 and Th9 cells: Progress and challenges. International Immunology. 2013;**25**:547-551

[71] Abadie V, Jabri B. IL-15: A central regulator of celiac disease immunopathology. Immunological Reviews. 2014;**260**:221-234

[72] Griffith JW, Sokol CL, Luster AD. Chemokines and chemokine receptors: Positioning cells for host defense and immunity. Annual Review of Immunology. 2014;**32**:659-702

[73] Delves PJ, Martin SJ, Burton DR, Roitt IM. Roitt's Essential Immunology. 12th ed. Oxford: Blackwell Publishing Limited; 2011

[74] Graves DT, Chemokines JY. A family of chemotactic cytokines. Critical Reviews in Oral Biology and Medicine: An Official Publication of the American Association of Oral Biologists. 1995;**6**:109-118

[75] Hamilton JA. Colony-stimulating factors in inflammation and autoimmunity. Nature Reviews Immunology. 2008;**8**:533-544

[76] Alam J, Jantan I, Bukhari SNA. Rheumatoid arthritis: Recent advances on its etiology, role of cytokines and pharmacotherapy. Biomedicine & Pharmacotherapy = Biomedecine & Pharmacotherapie. 2017;**92**:615-633

[77] Werth VP, Fiorentino D, Sullivan BA, Boedigheimer MJ, Chiu K, Wang C, et al. Brief report: Pharmacodynamics, safety, and clinical efficacy of AMG 811, a human anti-interferon-gamma antibody, in patients with discoid lupus erythematosus. Arthritis & Rheumatology. 2017;**69**:1028-1034

[78] Zhang YP, Wu J, Han YF, Shi ZR, Wang L. Pathogenesis of cutaneous lupus erythema associated with and without systemic lupus erythema. Autoimmunity Reviews. 2017;**16**:735-742

[79] Khan WA. Recombinant interferon alpha-2b is a high-affinity antigen for type 1 diabetes autoantibodies. Canadian Journal of Diabetes. 2017;**41**:217-223

[80] Alnek K, Kisand K, Heilman K, Peet A, Varik K, Uibo R. Increased blood levels of growth factors, proinflammatory cytokines, and Th17 cytokines in patients with newly diagnosed type 1 diabetes. PLoS One. 2015;**10**:e0142976

[81] Conigliaro P, Perricone C, Benson RA, Garside P, Brewer JM, Perricone R, et al. The type I IFN system in rheumatoid arthritis. Autoimmunity. 2010;**43**:220-225

[82] McInnes IB, Schett G. Cytokines in the pathogenesis of rheumatoid arthritis. Nature Reviews Immunology. 2007;**7**:429-442

[83] Khaibullin T, Ivanova V, Martynova E, Cherepnev G, Khabirov F, Granatov E, et al. Elevated levels of proinflammatory cytokines in cerebrospinal fluid of multiple sclerosis patients. Frontiers in Immunology. 2017;**8**:531

[84] Speeckaert R, Speeckaert M, De Schepper S, van Geel N. Biomarkers of disease activity in vitiligo: A systematic review. Autoimmunity Reviews. 2017;**16**:937-945

[85] Sanchez-Trujillo L, Vazquez-Garza E, Castillo EC, Garcia-Rivas G, Torre-Amione G. Role of adaptive immunity in the development and progression of heart failure: New evidence. Archives of Medical Research. 2017;**48**:1-11

Section 3

Autoantibodies and Cytokines in Different Diseases

Chapter 5

Autoantibodies in Viral Infections

Subuhi Sherwani, Mushtaq Ahmed Khan and
Mohammed Suliman Almogbel

Additional information is available at the end of the chapter

http://dx.doi.org/10.5772/intechopen.80471

Abstract

The immune system's ability to distinguish self from nonself is essential for initiating host defense against microbial antigens and protection of self-antigens from autoimmune-associated destruction. Virus infections have been implicated in the initiation of multiple human autoimmune diseases. This chapter aims to summarize the main principles for some specific viral infections and the subsequent production of autoantibodies resulting in the initiation, progression, and perpetuation of autoimmune diseases. Various mechanisms by which virus infections can induce autoimmune responses including molecular mimicry and epitope spreading are discussed with respect to these viruses, and evidence implicating virus infections in the pathogenesis of various human autoimmune diseases is reviewed. A better understanding of the viral origin of autoimmune diseases is an important step in the identification of high-risk patients as well as designing prevention and disruption strategies.

Keywords: autoimmune disease, autoimmunity, virus, Epstein-Barr virus, cytomegalovirus, hepatitis B virus

1. Introduction

An autoantibody is an antibody produced in response to a constituent of one's own cells or in other words produced against self-antigens such as nucleic acids, proteins, carbohydrates, lipids, and other multimolecular complexes. Autoantibodies may be organ-specific or systemic and are a characteristic feature of autoimmune disease (AD). Autoantibodies may also be produced as a result of different causes such as cancer, infection, or drug-related reactions [1]. The diagnosis and classification of autoimmune diseases (ADs) depends on serum autoantibodies out of which some specific ones have a prognostic significance and are thus used as markers to determine disease activity. Prior to clinical manifestation of an established AD, asymptomatic individuals may carry autoantibodies for many years. In such cases, the serological detection of these antibodies exhibits a strong predictive value [2–5].

2. Autoantibodies in viral disease

It is well established that there is often an association of transient, low-titer, polyspecific autoantibodies with common viral infections [6]. Autoantibodies may be detected in a variety of viral illnesses including hepatitis A, B, and C, parvovirus B19, enteroviruses, cytomegalovirus (CMV), and Epstein-Barr viruses (EBV) [1, 7–11]. Infectious agents have been implicated as an initial environmental trigger of AD in general, and in the induction of autoantibodies specifically [12–17]. It has been suggested that transient autoimmune responses are induced by acute viral infections in children and adults. Such responses may include generation of transient autoantibodies of typically low titer. The progression of such an immune state to an established autoimmune disease is rare [6, 18] as usually virally induced autoantibodies typically resolve with time. Hence, it may be difficult to differentiate autoimmune disease and self-limited illness.

Some of the commonly tested autoantibodies in viral infections include antinuclear antibodies (ANAs), antibodies directed against DNA, antibodies against proteins that bind to nucleic acids i.e. extractable nuclear antibodies (ENA), those directed against phospholipids, and anti-neutrophil cytoplasmic antibodies (ANCAs). In addition to these, the immune system may produce antibodies specific to certain tissues or organs (e.g., against hepatic, renal, gastric, intestinal, thyroid, pancreatic, muscular, testicular, dermatological, or neurological tissues). Also, the tendency of some viral infections to induce inflammatory responses in a variety of organ systems may also result in the development of autoimmune conditions. Hepatitis C and B virus, human immunodeficiency virus, parvovirus B19, cytomegalovirus, and Epstein-Barr virus appear to be associated with autoantibodies more commonly than other viruses.

2.1. Mechanism

The mechanisms responsible for the generation of autoantibodies as a result of viral infections remain unclear. A few proposed mechanisms include cross-reactivity between viral proteins and autoantigens [19], molecular mimicry [16, 17, 20], and the induction of apoptosis of virus-infected cells [21], all leading to the production of autoantibodies. Another theory suggests that autoantibodies are anti-idiotypic antibodies to antiviral antibodies [22]. However, molecular or antigenic mimicry between microbial proteins and self-components (i.e., proteins, carbohydrates, or DNA epitopes) remains the most likely mechanism of autoimmunity post viral infection [20, 23].

3. Viruses and autoimmunity

The existence of autoantibodies that do not induce tissue damage is known [19]; however, most of them are known to have clear pathogenic effects [24]. Pathogenic effects can vary from modulation of the biological activities such as cytotoxicity, phagocytosis and cell surface receptor binding, immune complex (consisting of viral antigen and antiviral antibodies)-mediated damage, and even lysis of the cell [24]. Although investigations into the relationship between viruses and the development of autoantibodies are ever continuing, we will focus on three different viruses that appear to be associated more commonly with autoimmunity than other viruses: Epstein-Barr virus (EBV), hepatitis B virus (HBV), and cytomegalovirus (CMV).

3.1. Epstein-Barr virus

Epstein-Barr virus (EBV) is a double-stranded DNA member of the gamma-herpesvirus family and is considered to be one of the most sinister members of the herpesvirus family. It usually infects young adults, adolescents, or children. EBV attacks and persists in B lymphocytes and based on viral antigen expression is known to exhibit up to four types of latency (latency 0–3). Upon reactivation from latent to lytic stage, the production of a large number of infectious virions leads to host cell lysis.

Autoantibodies can be detected during infectious mononucleosis, the symptomatic primary infection of EBV, and various other lymphoproliferative diseases caused by EBV [8, 25]. In some circumstances, it is known to cause many different systemic autoimmune diseases. However, the most widely understood relationship between this infamous infecting agent and another autoimmune disease is between EBV and systemic lupus erythematosus (SLE), which is often exhibited through a high prevalence of the virus in the sera of patients. Although several viral pathogens have been known to be associated with SLE, Epstein-Barr virus is considered to be one of the most important environmental factors in the etiology of this autoimmune disease. The serological correlation has been well established over the years [26] with modern diagnostic methods producing similar results [27].

Identification of a specific viral antigen that induces production of SLE-specific autoantibodies has proven to be difficult as the sera of patients with SLE can often exhibit more than 100 different autoantibodies [28]. Mechanisms responsible for EBV-associated SLE include molecular mimicry, bystander activation, and epitope spreading [29]. Molecular mimicry remains the most well-established method by which EBV infection is known to cause SLE [30]. EBV-associated autoimmunity is thus known to be caused by cross-reacting viral and endogenous proteins. It has also been well investigated that the immune response against EBV and EBV nuclear antigen 1 (EBNA-1) is different between patients with SLE and healthy controls. Whereas healthy controls maintain a partial humoral response and generally do not produce long-standing cross-reactive antibodies, patients with SLE exhibit humoral immune response to EBNA-1 with the generation of cross-reactive antibodies only in susceptible individuals [30]. Autoantibody complexes may also arise due to binding between SLE-specific autoantigens Sm and Ro and circulating anti-EBNA-1 antibodies, due to structural similarities. Furthermore, epitope spreading as a result of autoantibody complex accumulation will result on overt clinical disease [31, 32]. Apart from Ro and Sm, EBNA-1 may also elicit creation of anti-dsDNA, another SLE-associated autoantibody, also via molecular mimicry [32].

Another hypothesis suggests that B cells expressing the EBV-encoded protein latent membrane protein 2A bypasses normal tolerance checkpoints and induces hypersensitivity to Toll-like receptor stimulation, further activating anti-SmB cells through the B-cell receptor/Toll-like receptor pathway. Eventually, this leads to increased proliferation or differentiation of antibody-secreting cells or both [33]. A third hypothesis suggests that during primary infection, autoreactive B cells become infected by EBV and proliferate to become latently infected memory B cells. Since they express virus-encoded antiapoptotic molecules, these become resistant to normal B-cell homeostasis-associated apoptosis [34]. These impaired B cells activate autoreactive T cells which similarly fail to undergo apoptosis as they receive a costimulatory survival signal from infected B cells. The autoreactive T cells expand to produce cytokines, which recruit other inflammatory cells, resulting in target-organ damage and chronic autoimmune disease [35].

The association of EBV with rheumatoid arthritis is less clear. Patients with RA have higher levels of anti-EBV antibodies than healthy controls. Additionally, EBV-specific suppressor T-cell function is defective in rheumatoid arthritis, and patients with rheumatoid arthritis have a higher EBV load in peripheral blood lymphocytes. However, there is no clear evidence for the creation of rheumatoid arthritis-specific autoantibodies [36]. It has been proposed that EBV can, perhaps, play a role in the citrullination of autoantigens or the formation of autoantibodies such as anticyclic citrullinated peptide, but this theory remains to be proven [37].

Graves' disease is another autoimmune disease which is the most common cause of hyperthyroidism. It has been hypothesized by Nagata et al. that the reactivation of persisting Epstein-Barr virus in B lymphocytes induces differentiation of host B cells into plasma cells [38]. B cells infected with EBV possess thyrotropin receptor antibodies (TRAbs) on the surface of immunoglobulins (Igs) [39]. EBV reactivation induces these TRAb+EBV+ cells to produce TRAbs. Activation of B cells infected with the virus by polyclonal B cell activation leads to the production of Igs through plasma cell differentiation. This may be induced by EBV reactivation. EBV-LMP1 enables B cells to produce every isotype of Ig. Thus, it has been hypothesized that EBV rescues autoreactive B cells to produce autoantibodies, which contribute to the development and exacerbation of autoimmune diseases including Graves' disease [38].

3.2. Cytomegalovirus

Human cytomegalovirus (HCMV) or cytomegalovirus (CMV) is a large double-stranded DNA prototypic pathogenic member of the beta-subgroup of the herpesvirus family. Certain features attributed to the cytomegalovirus, like lytic replication in several different tissues, its lifelong persistence through periods of latency and reactivation, an extraordinarily large proteome, considerable manipulation of adaptive and innate immune systems, and its worldwide prevalence in human populations, make it a prominent candidate for involvement and exacerbation of autoimmune abnormalities [40]. Cytomegalovirus is known to be a leading cause of mental retardation and congenital hearing loss, and CMV infection is known to induce several autoimmune disorders in mice that resemble abnormalities in SLE [41]. It has also been implicated in the development and/or progression of SLE in humans [42]. Additionally, CMV has been associated with many other autoimmune diseases such as inflammatory bowel disease [43], diabetes mellitus [44, 45], systemic sclerosis [46], antiphospholipid syndrome [47, 48], and rheumatoid arthritis. The relationship between CMV infection and accelerated atherosclerosis [49, 50] is unclear, as conflicting data have been reported, and thus requires further investigation. A clear relationship between HCMV seroprevalence and disease has not been established. A higher prevalence of HCMV IgG antibodies would be expected in patients suffering from specific types of autoimmune diseases if HCMV is a causative agent for the onset of autoimmunity. The UL83-encoded pp65 matrix protein has been linked to autoantibodies in SLE patients [40]. Studies have found either higher HCMV-specific IgG titers [51] or higher frequencies of HCMV infection in patients with SLE [51, 52]. Moreover, in SLE patients with higher HCMV-specific IgG titers, more frequent autoantibodies could be detected [53, 54]. However, a clear cause-and-effect relationship between CMV infection and the creation of autoantibodies has yet to be ascertained. In a study of patients with SLE and some other autoimmune diseases such as Sjögren's syndrome, antiphospholipid syndrome, systemic sclerosis, biliary cirrhosis, polymyositis, or different types of vasculitis, a higher prevalence of CMV-associated IgM antibodies was detected [52]. The role of CMV in the pathogenesis of various autoimmune diseases requires further investigation.

3.3. Hepatitis B virus

Hepatitis B virus (HBV) is a small partially double-stranded circular DNA virus that replicates in the liver cells. This hepatotropic virus is classified in the Hepadnaviridae family. HBV remains one of the major causes of liver disease, varying in severity from person to person [53–56]. The most common autoimmune diseases associated with chronic HBV infection are membranous glomerulonephritis and systemic necrotizing vasculitis [57]. HBV uses active immune evasion strategies that target the adaptive response responsible for the elimination of HBV virus [55, 58]. CD4 T cells or helper T cells produce cytokines and are involved in the efficient development of effector cytotoxic CD8 T-cell antibody production by B cells. HBV-infected hepatocytes are cleared by CD8 T cells through both cytolytic and noncytolytic mechanisms, leading to a reduction in the levels of circulating virus. The B-cell antibody production neutralizes free viral particles and can also prevent infection or reinfection [55]. Liver injury during the acute and chronic phases of viral hepatitis may be caused by T-cell responses. HBV-specific $CD8^+$ T cells play a double role. On the one hand, the HBV-specific $CD8^+$ T cells are vital in the clearance and control of the virus, but on the other hand, when overall antiviral immunity is not robust enough to clear the viruses, liver tissue damage may occur through different pathways, including perforin-mediated cytotoxicity and Fas ligand/Fas-mediated apoptosis [59, 60]. Thus, liver damage in patients with chronic HBV infections may be a result of autoreactivity.

Antibodies against the asialoglycoprotein receptor-R have been reported in patients with chronic HBV [60]. The occurrence of antiasialoglycoprotein receptor-R antibodies in patients with moderate and severe chronic active hepatitis suggests that these antibodies are related to progressive liver damage development in patients with HBV infection rather than as simply a response to tissue damage. Either the host's immune response to virus-infected hepatocytes could result in liver damage [61] or this may be the effect of virus-induced apoptosis [21]. Autoantibodies produced as a direct result of this damage may be of various different kinds such as antiasialoglycoprotein receptor-R [60], antinuclear antibody [61], smooth muscle antibody [62, 63], antimitochondrial antibody [62], microsome antibody [62], rheumatoid factor [41], and proliferating cell nuclear antigen [61]. These autoantibodies bind to liver and kidney tissue and are directed against microsomal targets (expressed in estrogen receptor of these two organs) [64]. Further investigations are required to determine the cause-and-effect relationship between HBV and the generation of autoantibodies.

4. Conclusions

Viruses remain just one of the many etiological factors such as environmental stimuli, infection, genetic predisposition, cytokine activity, etc., which contribute to the development of autoimmune disease. Of the many mechanisms by which an infecting agent can induce an autoimmune reaction, molecular mimicry is probably one of the most common in viral-induced immunity. Over time, the development of chronic viral infections contributes to the development of a defective immune system, the accumulation of which gives rise to overt clinical illness. Thus, the study of infectious agents that play a role in the pathogenesis of this process is not only important to identify high-risk patients but also necessary in preventing the process of disease through medications. Prevention of such autoimmune abnormalities in general and virus-associated autoimmune phenomena in particular would be a great achievement in the field of autoimmunity.

Conflict of interest

The authors declare no conflict of interest.

Author details

Subuhi Sherwani*, Mushtaq Ahmed Khan and Mohammed Suliman Almogbel

*Address all correspondence to: susherwani@gmail.com

University of Hail, Hail, Saudi Arabia

References

[1] Schattner A. The origin of autoantibodies. Immunology Letters. 1987;**14**:143-153

[2] Shoenfeld Y, Blank M, Abu-Shakra M, Amital H, Barzilai O, Berkun Y. The mosaic of autoimmunity: Prediction, autoantibodies, and therapy in autoimmune diseases—2008. The Israel Medical Association Journal. 2008;**10**(1):13-19

[3] Harel M, Shoenfeld Y. Predicting and preventing autoimmunity, myth or reality? Annals of the New York Academy of Sciences. 2006;**1069**:322-345

[4] Lleo A, Invernizzi P, Gao B, Podda M, Gershwin ME. Definition of human autoimmunity—Autoantibodies versus autoimmune disease. Autoimmunity Reviews. 2010;**9**:A259-A266

[5] Scofield RH. Autoantibodies as predictors of disease. Lancet. 2004;**363**(9420):1544-1546

[6] Hansen KE, Arnason J, Bridges AJ. Autoantibodies and common viral illnesses. Seminars in Arthritis and Rheumatism. 1998;**27**:263-271

[7] Schattner A, Rager-Zisman B. Virus-induced autoimmunity. Reviews of Infectious Diseases. 1990;**12**:204-221

[8] Sutton RNP, Emond RTP, Thomas DB, Doniach D. The occurrence of autoantibodies in infectious mononucleosis. Clinical and Experimental Immunology. 1974;**17**:427-436

[9] Toh BH, Yeldiz A, Sotelo J, et al. Viral infections and IgM autoantibodies to cytoplasmic intermediate filaments. Clinical and Experimental Immunology. 1979;**37**:76-82

[10] Niwa Y, Sakane T, Kanoh T, et al. Transient autoantibodies with elevated complement levels in common viral diseases. Journal of Clinical & Laboratory Immunology. 1984;**13**: 183-188

[11] Vigeant P, Menard HA, Boire G. Chronic modulation of the autoimmune response following parvovirus B 19 infection. The Journal of Rheumatology. 1994;**21**:1165-1167

[12] Guilbert B, Dighiero G, Avrameas S. Naturally occurring antibodies against nine common antigens in human sera. Journal of Immunology. 1982;**128**:2779-2787

[13] Barzilai O, Ram M, Shoenfeld Y. Viral infection can induce the production of autoantibodies. Current Opinion in Rheumatology. 2007;**19**:636-643

[14] Kivity S, Agmon-Levin N, Blank M, Shoenfeld Y. Infections and autoimmunity—Friends or foes? Trends in Immunology. 2009;**30**:409-414

[15] Barzilai O, Sherer Y, Ram M, Izhaky D, Anaya JM, Shoenfeld Y. Epstein-Barr virus and cytomegalovirus in autoimmune diseases: Are they truly notorious? A preliminary report. Annals of the New York Academy of Sciences. 2007;**1108**:567-577

[16] Blank M, Barzilai O, Shoenfeld Y. Molecular mimicry and immunity. Clinical Reviews in Allergy and Immunology. 2007;**32**:111-118

[17] Agmon-Levin N, Blank M, Paz Z, Shoenfeld Y. Molecular mimicry in systemic lupus erythematosus. Lupus. 2009;**18**:1181-1185

[18] Denman AM, Rager-Zisman B. Viruses: The culprits of autoimmune diseases? In: Shoenfeld Y, Rose NR, editors. Infection and Autoimmunity. Amsterdam: Elsevier; 2004. pp. 123-153

[19] Yamamoto K. Possible mechanisms of autoantibody production and the connection of viral infections in human autoimmune diseases. The Tohoku Journal of Experimental Medicine. 1994;**173**:75-82

[20] Rose NR, Mackay IR. Molecular mimicry: A critical look at exemplary instances in human diseases. Cellular and Molecular Life Sciences. 2000;**57**:542-551

[21] Baumert TF, Thimme R, von Weizsacker F. Pathogenesis of hepatitis B virus infection. World Journal of Gastroenterology. 2007;**13**:82-90

[22] Plotz E. Autoantibodies are anti-idiotype antibodies to antiviral antibodies. Lancet. 1983;**2**: 824-826

[23] Peterson LK, Fujinami RS. Chapter 3: Molecular mimicry. In: Shoenfeld Y, Gershwin ME, Meroni PL, editors. Autoantibodies. 2nd ed. Oxford: Elsevier; 2007

[24] Cervera R, Shoenfeld Y. Pathogenic mechanisms and clinical relevance of autoantibodies. In: Shoenfeld Y, Gershwin ME, Meroni PL, editors. Autoantibodies. Amsterdam: Elsevier; 2007. pp. 29-35

[25] Nagata K, Okuno K, Ochi M, et al. Production of thyrotropin receptor antibodies in acute phase of infectious mononucleosis due to Epstein-Barr virus primary infection: A case report of a child. Springerplus. 2015;**4**:456. eCollection

[26] McClain MT, Harley JB, James JA. The role of Epstein-Barr virus in systemic lupus erythematosus. Frontiers in Bioscience. 2001;**6**:E137-E147

[27] Lu JJ, Chen DY, Hsieh CW, et al. Association of Epstein-Barr virus infection with systemic lupus erythematosus in Taiwan. Lupus. 2007;**16**:168-175

[28] Sherer Y, Gorstein A, Fritzler MJ, Shoenfeld Y. Autoantibody explosion in systemic lupus erythematosus: More than 100 different antibodies found in SLE patients. Seminars in Arthritis and Rheumatism. 2004;**34**:501-537

[29] Vista ES, Weisman MH, Ishimori ML, et al. Strong viral associations with SLE among Filipinos. Lupus Science & Medicine. 2017;**4**:e000214. DOI: 10.1136/lupus-2017-000214

[30] Poole BD, Scofield RH, Harley JB, James JA. Epstein-Barr virus and molecular mimicry in systemic lupus erythematosus. Autoimmunity. 2006;**39**:63-70

[31] Harley JB, Harley IT, Guthridge JM, James JA. The curiously suspicious: A role for Epstein-Barr virus in lupus. Lupus. 2006;**15**:768-777

[32] Sundar K, Jacques S, Gottlieb P, et al. Expression of the Epstein-Barr virus nuclear antigen-1 (EBNA-1) in the mouse can elicit the production of anti-dsDNA and anti-Sm antibodies. Journal of Autoimmunity. 2004;**23**:127-140

[33] Swanson-Mungerson M, Longnecker R. Epstein-Barr virus latent membrane protein 2A and autoimmunity. Trends in Immunology. 2007;**28**:213-218

[34] Wang H, Nicholas MW, Conway KL, et al. EBV latent membrane protein 2A induces autoreactive B cell activation and TLR hypersensitivity. Journal of Immunology. 2006; **177**:2793-2802

[35] Pender MP. Infection of autoreactive B lymphocytes with EBV, causing chronic autoimmune diseases. Trends in Immunology. 2003;**24**:584-588

[36] Balandraud N, Roudier J, Roudier C. Epstein-Barr virus and rheumatoid arthritis. Autoimmunity Reviews. 2004;**3**:362-367

[37] Costenbader KH, Karlson EW. Epstein-Barr virus and rheumatoid arthritis: Is there a link? Arthritis Research & Therapy. 2006;**8**:204

[38] Nagata K, Kumata K, Nakayama Y, et al. Epstein-Barr virus lytic reactivation activates B cells polyclonally and induces activation-induced cytidine deaminase expression: A mechanism underlying autoimmunity and its contribution to Graves' disease. Viral Immunology. 2017;**30**(3):240-249

[39] Tomer Y, Huber A. The etiology of autoimmune thyroid disease: A story of genes and environment. Journal of Autoimmunity. 2009;**32**:231-239

[40] Halenius A, Hengel H. Human cytomegalovirus and autoimmune disease. BioMed Research International. 2014;**2014**:15 pages, Article ID 472978. DOI: 10.1155/2014/472978

[41] Sekigawa I, Nawata M, Seta N, et al. Cytomegalovirus infection in patients with systemic lupus erythematosus. Clinical and Experimental Rheumatology. 2002;**20**:559-564

[42] Su BY, Su CY, Yu SF, Chen CJ. Incidental discovery of high systemic lupus erythematosus disease activity associated with cytomegalovirus viral activity. Medical Microbiology and Immunology. 2007;**196**:165-170

[43] Criscuoli V, Rizzuto MR, Cottone M. Cytomegalovirus and inflammatory bowel disease: Is there a link? World Journal of Gastroenterology. 2006;**12**:4813-4818

[44] Filippi C, von Herrath M. How viral infections affect the autoimmune process leading to type 1 diabetes. Cellular Immunology. 2005;**233**:125-132

[45] Roberts BW, Cech I. Association of type 2 diabetes mellitus and seroprevalence for cytomegalovirus. Southern Medical Journal. 2005;**98**:686-692

[46] Guiducci S, Giacomelli R, Tyndall A, Cerinic MM. Infection and systemic sclerosis. In: Shoenfeld Y, Rose NR, editors. Infection and Autoimmunity. Amsterdam: Elsevier; 2004. pp. 613-622

[47] Blank M, Asherson RA, Cervera R, Shoenfeld Y. Antiphospholipid syndrome infectious origin. Journal of Clinical Immunology. 2004;**24**:12-23

[48] Uthman I, Tabbarah Z, Gharavi AE. Hughes syndrome associated with cytomegalovirus infection. Lupus. 1999;**8**:775-777

[49] Nerheim PL, Meier JL, Vasef MA, et al. Enhanced cytomegalovirus infection in atherosclerotic human blood vessels. The American Journal of Pathology. 2004;**164**:589-600

[50] Degre M. Has cytomegalovirus infection any role in the development of atherosclerosis? Clinical Microbiology and Infection. 2002;**8**:191-195

[51] Esen BA, Yilmaz G, Uzun S, et al. Serologic response to Epstein-Barr virus antigens in patients with systemic lupus erythematosus: A controlled study. Rheumatology International. 2012;**32**(1):79-83

[52] Barzilai O, Sherer Y, Ram M, Izhaky D, Anaya J, Shoenfeld Y. EBV and CMV in autoimmune diseases. Are they truly notorious? A preliminary report. Annals of the New York Academy of Sciences. 2007;**1108**:567-577

[53] Palafox S'anchez CA, Satoh M, Chan EK, et al. Reduced IgG anti-small nuclear ribonucleoprotein autoantibody production in systemic lupus erythematosus patients with positive IgM anti-cytomegalovirus antibodies. Arthritis Research & Therapy. 2009;**11**(1):R27

[54] Shepard CW, Simard EP, Finelli L, et al. Hepatitis B virus infection: Epidemiology and vaccination. Epidemiologic Reviews. 2006;**28**:112-125

[55] Bertoletti A, Gehring AJ. The immune response during hepatitis B virus infection. The Journal of General Virology. 2006;**87**:1439-1449

[56] Huang CF, Lin SS, Ho YC, et al. The immune response induced by hepatitis B virus principal antigens. Cellular & Molecular Immunology. 2006;**3**:97-106

[57] Acay A, Demir K, Asik G, Tunay H, Acarturk G. Assessment of the frequency of autoantibodies in chronic viral hepatitis. Pakistan Journal of Medical Sciences. 2015;**31**(1):150-154. DOI: 10.12669/pjms.311.6053

[58] Wieland SF, Chisari FV. Stealth and cunning: Hepatitis B and hepatitis C viruses. Journal of Virology. 2005;**79**:9369-9380

[59] Ichiki Y, He XS, Shimoda S, et al. T cell immunity in hepatitis B and hepatitis C virus infection: Implications for autoimmunity. Autoimmunity Reviews. 2005;**4**:82-95

[60] McFarlane BM, Bridger CB, Smith HM, et al. Autoimmune mechanisms in chronic hepatitis B and delta virus infections. European Journal of Gastroenterology & Hepatology. 1995;**7**:615-621

[61] Tzang BS, Chen TY, Hsu TC, et al. Presentation of autoantibody to proliferating cell nuclear antigen in patients with chronic hepatitis B and C virus infection. Annals of the Rheumatic Diseases. 1999;**58**:630-634

[62] Zachou K, Liaskos C, Christodoulou DK, et al. Anticardiolipin antibodies in patients with chronic viral hepatitis are independent of beta2-glycoprotein I cofactor or features of antiphospholipid syndrome. European Journal of Clinical Investigation. 2003;**33**:161-168

[63] Invernizzi P. Antinuclear antibodies: General introduction. In: Shoenfeld Y, Gershwin ME, Meroni PL, editors. Autoantibodies. Amsterdam: Elsevier; 2007. pp. 129-133

[64] Strassburg CP, Manns MP. Liver cytosol antigen type I autoantibodies, liver kidney microsomal autoantibodies, and liver microsomal autoantibodies. In: Shoenfeld Y, Gershwin ME, Meroni PL, editors. Autoantibodies. Amsterdam: Elsevier; 2007. pp. 463-471

Chapter 6

Autoantibodies and Cytokines in Pathogenesis of Rheumatoid Arthritis

Mohd Wajid Ali Khan and Wahid Ali Khan

Additional information is available at the end of the chapter

http://dx.doi.org/10.5772/intechopen.82265

Abstract

Rheumatoid arthritis (RA) is an autoimmune disorder in which increased autoantibody production and enhanced secretion of pro-inflammatory cytokines are the hallmark of the disease. A strictly controlled balance of antibody production and proinflammatory cytokines is the key to the healthy state. A slight tilt in this balance causes proinflammatory diseases. In RA there is an increased production of autoantibodies such as rheumatoid factor (RF) and anti-citrullinated protein antibody (ACPA), anti-cartilage type II antibodies, and etc., which have a prominent clinical significance. Furthermore, there is increased secretion of proinflammatory cytokines such as tumor necrosis factor-α (TNFα), interleukin-6 (IL-6), interleukin-1 (IL-1) which have an impact of great magnitude on the RA disease progression and severity. A better understanding of the mechanism of autoantibody production and secretion of cytokines together with crosstalk between immune cells and cytokines can provide us a better insight into the disease pathogenesis as well disease prognosis and management.

Keywords: rheumatoid arthritis, autoantibodies, cytokines, proinflammatory, pathogenesis

1. Introduction

Autoimmunity arises as a result of failure of immune self-tolerance. The condition may involve both T and B cells however it has been found that in most autoimmune diseases, T cells play a pivotal role in both dysregulation and autoimmune aggression, but autoantibodies are also widely produced by B cells. Such autoantibodies play a key pathogenic role in diseases such as autoimmune hemocytopenias, Grave's disease, rheumatoid arthritis, type 1 diabetes and systemic lupus erythemathosus (SLE). Similarly, autoantibodies are also found in other diseases, where although they may play a minor pathogenic role, but can be used as valuable diagnostic markers [1–7].

Furthermore, in addition to T cells and autoantibodies, cytokines also play a pivotal role in development of the autoimmune response. Proinflammatory cytokines have significant involvement in autoimmune associated damage. This chapter aims to discuss the involvement of autoantibodies and cytokines in the pathogenesis of RA.

Immune system has the capacity to mount an immune response against virtually all foreign molecules as well as self. However, several mechanisms exist within the human system that prevent or subdue the response to self-antigens. The immune system has developed a series of checks and balances that enable it to distinguish dangerous signals from harmless ones and allow it to respond to foreign or non-self-antigens. When these mechanisms undergo a breakdown or are overridden, a response directed against self-antigen can occur, resulting in autoimmune reactions and/or autoimmune diseases [8].

RA is a complex chronic disease, primarily affects the lining of the synovial joints and can cause progressive disability, premature death, and socioeconomic burdens. The clinical manifestations of symmetrical joint involvement include arthralgia, swelling, redness, and even limiting the range of motion [9].

Autoantibodies have been associated with human pathologies for a long time, particularly with autoimmune diseases. RA is more frequent in females as compared to males [10]. Organ specific autoimmune diseases involve single or multiple autoantigens. In RA, presence of various autoantibodies such as RF and ACPA, and anti-cartilage type II antibodies in serum and synovial fluid have long been associated with RA severity [11].

The pathological hallmarks of synovitis in rheumatoid arthritis include the proliferation of resident synovial fibroblasts, new blood vessel formation and the recruitment of a wide range of leukocytes including B and T lymphocytes, monocytes/macrophages and mast cells; in turn this leads to synovial hypertrophy and the invasion of cartilage and bone by activated inflammatory tissue. Cytokines are fundamental orchestrators of the development and maintenance of this lesion [12]. RA disorder is a multifactorial disorder other than autoantibodies there are many other important factors involved such as proinflammatory cytokines such as TNF-α, IL-6 and IL-1 are key mediators of cell migration and inflammation in RA [13]. Cartilage degradation in RA occurs when TNF-α, IL-1 and IL-6 activate synoviocytes, resulting in the secretion of matrix metalloproteinases (MMPs), cathepsins and mast cell proteinases into the synovial fluid [14, 15]. Cytokines also activate chondrocytes, leading to the direct release of additional MMPs into the cartilage [14, 15].

Although the availability of advanced drugs and treatment regimes, however the complete remission of the disease is still not achieved. This chapter shed light on the complex network of the autoantibodies and proinflammatory cytokines as immune responses in the RA disease pathogenesis and the development of bio-therapeutics used in RA disorder.

http://dx.doi.org/10.5772/intechopen.82265

2. Autoantibodies in RA

Several studies have been demonstrated that levels of disease-related biomarkers (such as RF and antibodies to citrullinated protein antigen, as well as secretory phospholipase A2, C-reactive protein (CRP), glycated HSA, and multiple cytokines/chemokines) may be elevated prior to the onset of symptomatic rheumatoid arthritis [16–24].

These findings suggest that there is a substantial "preclinical" period of RA, during which detectable immunologic and inflammatory changes are occurring that are related to disease development. These increased levels of RA related autoantibodies in preclinical RA may be highly specific for early RA detection [18, 19]. There is a great hope that these autoantibodies may be used to predict which currently asymptomatic individuals are at sufficiently high risk for future RA that they may be targeted with preventive therapies.

2.1. Rheumatoid factors

The RA is associated with systemic autoimmunity as evidenced by the presence of serum and synovial fluid autoantibodies. The first autoantibody to be described in RA was the rheumatoid factor (RF) by Waaler in 1940 [25], and it was later found to be directed to the Fc region of IgG. It is well characterized, although its exact origin still remains unclear. Typically, RF is of IgM isotype, but IgG and IgA may also occur. IgM RFs are the major RF species in RA and are detected in 60–80% of RA patients [26]. In the past, RF levels were determined by classical agglutination reactions; however, sensitivities and specificities depended on the type of test (e.g., latex fixation test, or Waaler-Rose test using sheep erythrocytes). RF levels were also determined by nephelometry [27]. RF has been observed in many other autoimmune diseases, such as, in systemic lupus erythematosus, mixed connective tissue disease and primary Sjogren syndrome, as well as in non-autoimmune conditions, such as in chronic infections and old age [26]. RF specificity to RA is increased at high titers (e.g., IgM RF > 50 IU/ml) and with IgA isotypes [26, 28, 29]. High titer RF and IgA isotypes are also associated with radiologic erosion, extra-articular manifestations and thus, poorer outcomes [26, 28, 30, 31]. The association between high titer RF status and a poor prognosis indicates that RF may have a role in the pathogenesis of RA. The functions of RFs under normal physiological conditions were observed as (i) enhancement of immune complex clearance by increasing its avidity and size, (ii) aiding B cells in uptake of immune complex through efficient antigen presentation to T cells, and (iii) facilitation of complement fixation by binding to IgG containing immune complexes [32–34]. RFs with high affinity and high-titer in synovial fluid of RA patients are considered to exert pathogenic functions and to enhance inflammation and antigen trapping in joints. However, no clear evidence yet suggests that RFs are involved in the initial events triggering the disease process of RA. In fact, it is understood that they may themselves be triggered by RA. Somatic mutations accumulates in RA and the presence of isotype switching indicate that RF production is T-cell driven, although T cells infiltrate RA synovium [35] and contain autoreactive clones [36], which were polyclonal and lack specificity for any particular autoantigen [36, 37]. T-cell clones reactive with autologous IgG were not detected in

RA patients as yet. Additionally, the function of RF expressing B cells to take up immune complexes and present trapped antigens to T cells may allow these cells to bypass the need for specific T cell help and eventually lead to emergence of autoreactive T cells capable of triggering RF synthesis in the absence of an external antigen [38].

2.2. Anti-citrullinated proteins antibodies (ACPA) in RA

Some other names used to describe ACPA are anti-keratin, antiperinuclear factor antibodies, antifilaggrin antibodies, or anti-Sa [39]. ACPA have been associated with human pathology [40] as well as preclinical disease [16, 18, 41]. Latest ELISA assays, exhibited higher specificity (~98%) and sensitivity between 40 and 76% (depending on disease stage) [42]. Recently proved that there is a potential association of ACPA with conditions like psoriatic arthritis [43], periodontitis [44], and osteoarthritis [45]. The key difference between ELISA assays was in the antigens used to detect ACPA. Thus, the diagnostic value of ACAP was established by demonstrating the significance of using appropriate citrullinated peptide [39, 46, 47]. Consequentially, a highly sensitive noncommercial ELISA, based on protein targets identified as reactive with ACPA in synovial tissue such as alpha and beta fibrinogen was therefore developed [48]. The positivity of ACPA for one or both to these two citrullinated peptides covered all reactivity in RA sera [49].

Citrullinated peptides are generated in response to a posttranslational modification mediated by peptidyl-arginine deiminase (PAD) enzymes. Multiple antibody isotypes including IgG, IgA, and IgM directed against these citrullinated peptides are detected in RA [50]. Citrullinated proteins are present in the synovial fluid of inflamed RA joints, exhibiting that ACPA could bind to these antigens in the joint and possibly increase local inflammation [51]. A protein that is commonly targeted by ACPA is Vimentin. In collagen-induced arthritis, mouse models passive transfer of ACPA cannot cause synovitis, although it can worsen preexistent synovitis [52]. Therefore, it is suggested that multiple events are necessary for the development of RA.

ACPA causes inflammation via binding to Fc receptors or complement activation. Autoantibodies are usually glycoproteins that means both Fc and Fab region of the antibody bind to the carbohydrate chains, which is essential for immune effector functions. Compared to IgG antibodies, the Fc region of ACPA has a lower level of galactosylation and sialylation against recall antigens [53]. The decreased sialylation of IgG in immune complexes can drive osteoclastogenesis, both *in vitro* and *in vivo*, through altered FcγR signaling. Moreover, it has been found that RA patients with low levels of ACPA-IgG Fc sialylation displayed lower bone volumes and trabecula numbers [54]. Thus, disease pathophysiology could be influenced by the specific Fc glycan signature of ACPA.

2.3. Autoantibodies against type II collagen

Type II collagen (CII) are abundantly present in joint cartilage [55]. Native CII protein consists of a triple-helix structure containing three identical α chains. The collagen fibrils contribute to cartilage integrity by resisting stretching forces caused by hydrophilic proteoglycan molecules in extracellular matrix of articular cartilage, [56]. The degradation of CII leads to the degeneration of cartilage and consequent loss of function in RA patients [57]. Denaturation of CII also causes separation of α chains and loss of antigenic sites (epitopes) present in the molecule which are altered due to the disruption of its three dimensional structure [58]. Autoantibodies to both, native and denatured CII, have been reported in RA [59–62]. Varying levels of anti-CII antibodies were detected in the same patient at different times and also between patients, suggesting that these antibodies might be associated with specific events during arthritis development.

Increased anti-CII antibody levels may degrade CII molecules leading to acute inflammation which is mediated by anti-CII antibody containing surface-bound immune complexes (ICs) [60], which activates complement system activation and enhanced the production of proinflammatory cytokines (TNFα, IL-1β and IL-8) [63], which leads to the inflammation of the joints and hence cartilage damage. Antibodies have been detected against major CII epitopes at the site of inflammation, serum and synovial fluid samples from RA patients, supporting the concept of an increased local immune response to CII in the joints [61].

CII is found to be arthritogenic in animals and an injection of native CII in adjuvant induces collagen-induced arthritis (CIA) characterized by antibodies to CII and inflammatory polyarthritis [64]. Variability in expression of arthritis is linked to the expression of particular class II major histocompatibility (MHC) alleles [65] and also depends on an intact immune system. For example, B cell deficient animals [66] or complement deficient ones [67] are protected. Moreover, monoclonal antibodies (mAb) to CII derived from mice with CIA can induce collagen antibody-induced arthritis (CAIA) in naïve mice. CAIA is a condition characterized by inflammation, formation of pannus and erosions of bone similar to that observed in RA [68]. This model disease does not require the help pf T cells and has proven to be an informative model to better understand how antibodies lead to development of arthritis. Not only is arthritis not MHC-restricted, but it can be induced in most strains of mice and represents a model of the effector arm of CIA. However, it depends on the specificity of the antibodies used. A triplet of arginine-glycine-hydrophobic acids, is a common amino acid motif, shared by these arthritogenic mAb, which recognize epitopes on CII. These map to surface-exposed regions on the collagen fibrils that are accessible for antibody binding [68]. These epitopes are conserved, and are also recognized by antibodies from rats [69–71] and from humans with RA [70, 72]. Amino acid arginine molecules are present on the surface of the major epitopes on the collagen fibrils can also become citrullinated [73] and mAb reactive with these citrullinated epitopes may be arthritogenic themselves, or induce more severe arthritis when injected with subclinical doses of anti-CII [74]. Antibodies to major CII epitopes could be useful as markers for the biomonitoring of joint destruction in some patients.

3. Role of cytokines in RA

The network of cytokine in the RA disease is very complex system, with a numerous of cytokines showing pleiotropic actions and many different targets. This network can be divided in two groups, the pro-inflammatory and anti-inflammatory cytokines. Controlling the balance between these two groups is considered as an important therapeutic goal. This chapter provide an important role of TNF-α in the pathogenesis of RA, leading to the first clinical trials of a biological therapeutic in this disease. Other than TNF-α we address other cytokines such as IL-1, IL-6 and IL-23 that might play a role in the disease, together with selected cytokines that bind a receptor containing the common γ-chain (γc) [75].

3.1. TNF-α

TNF-α is a proinflammaotory cytokine and played a key role in RA with its potential to degrade cartilage [76] and bone [77] *in vitro*. It has been shown in an experiment that dissociated RA synovial mononuclear cell cultures that TNF-α as well as other proinflammatory cytokines (IL-1, IL-6, GM-CSF, and IL-8) [78–81] were produced in a five-day culture [82, 83]. When the activity of TNF-α was blocked in these cultures, the spontaneous production of both IL-1 protein and IL1B mRNA was remarkably decreased and IL-1 bioactivity was neutralized [82]. This is the evidence that the secretion of all these cytokines is a network and controlled by hierarchy of their expressions.

Soluble TNF receptors are found in high concentrations in the synovial fluid and serum of patient with RA [84]. RA patients are found to have high levels of TNF-α in the synovial fluid. This plays an important role in inflammation and joint destruction, both of which are hallmarks of RA. Anti-TNF-α therapy induces a shift in the cytokine equilibrium producing more anti-inflammatory cytokines. Studies have demonstrated dramatic improvement in synovial inflammation in RA patients after treatment with neutralizing anti-TNF-α Abs or soluble TNF receptors. They also suggest decreased joint destruction after treatment with IL-1Ra [85].

In a first clinical trial of a TNF-α blocking agent for the treatment of 20 active RA patients were initiated. Infliximab (Remicade), a chimeric antibody specific for human TNF-α was used. Signs and symptoms of the RA disease were substantially reduced with the treatment with infliximab together with decreased levels of CRP in the serum [86]. Other multicentric placebo-controlled trials were also confirmed the therapeutic efficacy of infliximab when coadministrated with methotrexate. This led eventually to FDA approval of the drug for the treatment of RA [87, 88]. After two-year of clinical trial, it was observed that there was a retardation or arrest of both joint space narrowing and bone erosion due to infliximab and methotrexate therapy [89]. There were two other drugs etanercept (Enbrel) and adalimumab (Humira) which are functioned as TNF-α blockers were used in the treatment of RA.

TNF-α is now considered as controlling a wide variety of effector functions relevant to the pathogenesis of RA, including endothelial cell activation and chemokines production which causes accumulation of leukocytes [90]; osteoclast and chondrocyte activation, promoting articular destruction. These all are RA disease pathogenesis spectrum which explains the broad role of TNF-α blockade in patients. Further, improved therapies targeting TNF-α would be a potential therapeutics for the treatment of RA.

3.2. Interleukin-1

Each member of the IL-1 family binds with high affinity to specific receptors. Binding of IL-1α or IL-1β to type I IL-1 receptors (IL-1RI), can is enhanced by an accessory protein, IL-1R-AcP, leads to intracellular signal transduction and regulation of gene expression and hence cellular responses [91]. The extent of response of IL-1β in the rheumatoid joint depends on a few factors such as (1) IL-1β and IL-1Rα have similar affinity for IL-1RI on synoviocytes, chondrocytes and other cells and hence, the relative concentrations of IL-1β and IL-1Rα are important in determining the level of cell activation and biological responses, (2) a greater number of IL-1RII reduces the amount of IL-1β and IL-1Rα, that is available for binding to IL-1RI. Similarly, soluble IL-1 receptors found in synovial fluid and in the circulation also decrease the amount of these cytokines available to interact with IL-1RI. The response of IL-1β, as well as to other proinflammatory cytokines, is regulated by various anti-inflammatory and immunomodulatory cytokines, including IL-4, IL-10, IL-11, IL-13 and transforming growth factor-β [91, 92].

IL1 causes inflammatory cells to move into the joints and the synovium in RA patients. An unspecified antigenic trigger is thought to activate the production of IL1 in joints by macrophages (lymphocytes, monocytes and transformed fibroblasts) [54, 93]. These cells secrete proteases and proteoglycans as cellular signals, that may result in pannus formation, which accumulates in the joints. Destructive enzymes can enter and destroy cartilage and ultimately degrade and erode bone. Importantly, specifically blocking IL1 is a targeted, rational treatment against the destructive functions of IL1 in RA [54, 94].

Evidence from experimental studies in animal models of arthritis and from an x randomized controlled trials in patients with RA indicates that IL-1 plays an important role in RA pathogenesis, and that IL-1 inhibition with anakinra is effective in slowing further radiographic progression of the disease and hence models significantly reduces bone erosions and cartilage degradation [14]. It is important to elucidate that, whether slowing radiographic progression with these biological therapies will significantly improve long-term outcomes in RA.

3.3. Interleukin-6

IL-6 is an essential and multifunctional proinflammatory cytokine of the immune system and could be a key mediator for the development of many chronic inflammatory or autoimmune diseases including RA [95, 96].

It is well established that increased levels of autoantibodies are the characteristics of autoimmune RA and hence decreased levels of antibody producing B cells are might have a therapeutic efficacy demonstrates the impact of B-cell activity on synovial inflammation and joint damage. IL-6 stimulates B cells to differentiate into plasma cells to produce immunoglobulins [97]. IL-6 induces B-cell differentiation [98] and it has been established that B-cells induced antibody production [99].

Neutrophils can be directly activated by IL-6 through membrane-bound receptor IL-6R, which in turn help inflammation and joint destruction through the secretion of proteolytic enzymes and reactive oxygen intermediates [100]. An *in vitro* study with fibroblasts from patients with RA showed the role of IL-6 in actively encourage the recruitment of neutrophil by activated fibroblasts. Although untreated fibroblasts were able to recruit neutrophils, it was found that the recruitment was inhibited in the presence of anti-IL-6 antibody [101].

Osteoclasts are multinucleated cells formed by the fusion of mononuclear progenitors of the monocyte and macrophage family. These cells populate the synovial membranes of RA patients and are concentrated in bones [102, 103]. Macrophage derived osteoclastogenesis requires the presence of macrophage colony-stimulating factor. It results from the interaction of the RANK and the RANK ligand (RANKL) [102]. RANKL expression is regulated by pro-inflammatory cytokines such as TNF-α, IL-1, IL-6 and IL-17 [103].

The principal cause of bone erosion is the pannus, which is found at the interface with cartilage and bone. Angiogenesis is an important process in the formation and maintenance of pannus [104]. Vascular endothelial growth factor (VEGF), is an important angiogenic mediator which promotes the migration and proliferation of endothelial cells, as well as inducing vascular permeability and mediating inflammation [105]. Increased levels of VEGF correlate with disease activity in RA patients [106]. IL-6 in the presence of sIL-6R increased VEGF levels in cultured synovial fibroblasts from RA patients and anti-IL-6R antibody significantly reduced VEGF concentration [107].

Blocking antibodies were used with other agents as a combinational therapeutics for the treatment of RA. A humanized anti-IL-6R monoclonal antibody, tocilizumab (TCZ), used in a first clinical trial was conducted in patients with established RA [108]. A total of 45 patients were randomized to receive a single intravenous infusion of TCZ of 0.1, 1, 5, 10 mg/kg or placebo. Patients in the 5 and 10 mg/kg arms showed rapidly improvement in disease activity. CRP normalized after treatment in the 5 and 10 mg/kg treated patients confirming IL-6 as the dominant cytokine in generating the acute-phase response in patients with RA. Another, double-blind, placebo-controlled trial in 164 RA patients was conducted and demonstrates that the clinical response was maintained with repeated dosing of TCZ monotherapy [109]. A European study CHARISMA, examined the combinational effect of TCZ with methotrexate (MTX). In the study of 359 RA patients with partial response to MTX, it was found that TCZ was efficacious as monotherapy or in combination with MTX although the latter appeared to enhance the benefit of TCZ [110]. There were many other clinical trials and studies that ensures the use of TCZ alone or in combinational therapies such as MTX results in sustained improvement in physical function and reduced radiographic joint damage in RA [111–117].

4. Conclusion

RA is a complex disease that develops through a series of events often referred to as disease continuum. It is an autoimmune and inflammatory disease that can be further aggravated with the increased production and secretion of autoantibodies (RF ACPA, anti-cartilage type II antibodies) and the secretion of proinflammatory cytokines (TNF, IL-1, IL-6). With a better knowledge and understanding of the crosstalk between the molecules involved in RA disease pathogenesis, it would be easier to identify better markers for RA disease as well as design and administer specific and efficient therapeutics that can control RA pathogenesis and deliver long term and permanent remission of the disease.

Author details

Mohd Wajid Ali Khan[1]* and Wahid Ali Khan[2]

*Address all correspondence to: wajidkhan11@gmail.com

1 Department of Clinical Laboratory Sciences, College of Applied Medical Sciences, University of Hail, Ha'il, Kingdom of Saudi Arabia

2 Department of Clinical Biochemistry, College of Medicine, King Khalid University, Abha, Kingdom of Saudi Arabia

References

[1] Özen S, Berk Ö, Şimşek DG, Darcan S. Clinical course of Hashimoto's thyroiditis and effects of levothyroxine therapy on the clinical course of the disease in children and adolescents. Journal of Clinical Research in Pediatric Endocrinology. 2011;**3**:192-197

[2] McKee A, Peyerl F. TSI assay utilization: Impact on costs of Graves'hyperthyroidism diagnosis. The American Journal of Managed Care. 2012;**18**:e1-e14

[3] Sblattero D, Berti I, Trevisiol C, Marzari R, Tommasini A, Bradbury A, et al. Human recombinant tissue transglutaminase ELISA: An innovative diagnostic assay for celiac disease. The American Journal of Gastroenterology. 2000;**95**:1253-1257

[4] Sultan Alouffi S, Sherwani S, Al-Mogbel MS, Sherwani MKA, Khan MWA. Depression and smoking augment the production of circulating autoantibodies against glycated HSA in rheumatoid arthritis patients. International Archives of Allergy and Immunology. 2018;**29**:1-11

[5] Khan MWA, Qadrie ZL, Khan WA. Antibodies against gluco-oxidatively modified human serum albumin detected in diabetes-associated complications. International Archives of Allergy and Immunology. 2010;**153**:207-214

[6] Khan, Sherwani S, Khan WA, Moinuddin, Ali R. Characterization of hydroxyl radical modified GAD65: A potential autoantigen in type 1 diabetes. Autoimmunity. 2009; **42**(2):150-158

[7] Khan MWA, Banga K, Mashal SN, Khan WA. Detection of autoantibodies against reactive oxygen species modified glutamic acid decarboxylase-65 in type 1 diabetes associated complications. BMC Immunology. 2011;**12**:19

[8] Khan FH. Autoimmunity and Autoimmune Diseases. The Elements of Immunology. India: Pearson Education; 2009

[9] Guo Q, Wang Y, Xu D, Nossent J, Pavlos NJ, Xu J. Rheumatoid arthritis: Pathological mechanisms and modern pharmacologic therapies. Bone Research. 2018;**6**:15

[10] Silman AJ, Pearson JE. Epidemiology and genetics of rheumatoid arthritis. Arthritis Research. 2002;**4**(3):S265-S272

[11] McInnes IB, Schett G. The pathogenesis of rheumatoid arthritis. The New England Journal of Medicine. 2011;**365**(23):2205-2219

[12] Ridgley LA, Anderson AE, Pratt AG. What are the dominant cytokines in early rheumatoid arthritis? Current Opinion in Rheumatology. 2018;**30**(2):207-214

[13] Smolen JS, Aletaha D, Koeller M, Weisman MH, Emery P. New therapies for treatment of rheumatoid arthritis. Lancet. 2007;**370**:1861-1874

[14] Strand V, Kavanaugh AF. The role of interleukin-1 in bone resorption in rheumatoid arthritis. Rheumatology. 2004;**43**(Suppl. 3):iii10-iii16

[15] Johnson LL, Dyer R, Hupe DJ. Matrix metalloproteinases. Current Opinion in Chemical Biology. 1998;**2**:466-471

[16] Kurki P, Aho K, Palosuo T, Heliovaara M. Immunopathology of rheumatoid arthritis: Antikeratin antibodies precede the clinical disease. Arthritis and Rheumatism. 1992;**35**:914-917

[17] Aho K, Palosuo T, Heliovaara M, Knekt P, Alha P, von Essen R. Antifilaggrin antibodies within "normal" range predict rheumatoid arthritis in a linear fashion. The Journal of Rheumatology. 2000;**27**:2743-2746

[18] Rantapaa-Dahlqvist S, de Jong BA, Berglin E, Hallmans G, Wadell G, Stenlund H, et al. Antibodies against cyclic citrullinated peptide and IgA rheumatoid factor predict the development ofrheumatoid arthritis. Arthritis and Rheumatism. 2003;**48**:2741-2749

[19] Nielen MM, van Schaardenburg D, Reesink HW, van, de Stadt RJ, van, der Horst-Bruinsma IE, de Koning MH, et al. Specific autoantibodies precede the symptoms of rheumatoid arthritis: A study of serial measurements in blood donors. Arthritis and Rheumatism. 2004;**50**:380-386

[20] Nielen MM, van Schaardenburg D, Reesink HW, Twisk JW, van, de Stadt RJ, van, der Horst-Bruinsma IE, et al. Increased levels of C-reactive protein in serum from blood donors before the onset of rheumatoid arthritis. Arthritis and Rheumatism. 2004; **50**:2423-2427

[21] Jorgensen KT, Wiik A, Pedersen M, Hedegaard CJ, Vestergaard BF, Gislefoss RE, et al. Cytokines, autoantibodies and viral antibodies in premorbid and postdiagnostic sera from patients with rheumatoid arthritis: Case-control study nested in a cohort of Norwegian blood donors. Annals of the Rheumatic Diseases. 2008;**67**:860-866

[22] Shadick NA, Cook NR, Karlson EW, Ridker PM, Maher NE, Manson JE, et al. C-reactive protein in the prediction of rheumatoid arthritis in women. Archives of Internal Medicine. 2006;**166**:2490-2494

[23] Kokkonen H, Soderstrom I, Rocklov J, Hallmans G, Lejon K, Rantapaa Dahlqvist S. Up-regulation of cytokines and chemokines predates the onset of rheumatoid arthritis. Arthritis and Rheumatism. 2010;**62**:383-391

[24] Karlson EW, Chibnik LB, Tworoger SS, Lee IM, Buring JE, Shadick NA, et al. Biomarkers of inflammation and development of rheumatoid arthritis in women from two prospective cohort studies. Arthritis and Rheumatism. 2009;**60**:641-652

[25] Waaler E. On the occurrence of a factor in human serum activating the specific agglutination of sheep red corpuscles. Acta Pathologica et Microbiologica Scandinavica. 1940;**17**:172-188

[26] Nell VP, Machold KP, Stamm TA, Eberl G, Heinzl H, Uffmann M, et al. Autoantibody profiling as early diagnostic and prognostic tool for rheumatoid arthritis. Annals of the Rheumatic Diseases. 2005;**64**:1731-1736

[27] Roberts-Thomson PJ, Wernick RM, Ziff M. Quantitation of rheumatoid factor by laser nephelometry. Rheumatology International. 1982;**2**:17-20

[28] Jo'nsson T, Steinsson K, Jo'nsson H, Geirsson AJ, Thorsteinsson J, Valdimarsson H. Combined elevation of IgM and IgA rheumatoid factor has high diagnostic specificity for rheumatoid arthritis. Rheumatology International. 1998;**18**:119-122

[29] Jo'nsson T, Arinbjarnarson S, Thorsteinsson J, Steinsson K, Geirsson AJ, Jo'nsson H, et al. Raised IgA rheumatoid factor (RF) but not IgM RF or IgG RF is associated with extra-articular manifestations in rheumatoid arthritis. Scandinavian Journal of Rheumatology. 1995;**24**:372-375

[30] Jorgensen C, Legouffe MC, Bologna C, Brochier J, Sany J. IgA isotype rheumatoid factor in rheumatoid arthritis: Clinical implications. Clinical and Experimental Rheumatology. 1996;**14**:301-304

[31] Pai S, Päi L, Birkenfeldt R. Correlation of serum IgA rheumatoid factor levels with disease severity in rheumatoid arthritis. Scandinavian Journal of Rheumatology. 1998;**27**:252-256

[32] Van Snick JL, Van Roost E, Markowetz B, Cambiaso CL, Masson PL. Enhancement by IgM rheumatoid factor of in vitro ingestion by macrophages and in vivo clearance of aggregated IgG or antigen-antibody complexes. European Journal of Immunology. 1978;**8**:279-285

[33] Brown PB, Nardella FA, Mannik M. Human complement activation by self-associated IgG rheumatoid factors. Arthritis and Rheumatism. 1982;**25**:1101-1107

[34] Tighe H, Chen PP, Tucker R, Kipps TJ, Roudier J, Jirik FR, et al. Function of B cells expressing a human immunoglobulin M rheumatoid factor autoantibody in transgenic mice. The Journal of Experimental Medicine. 1993;**177**:109-118

[35] Firestein GS. Rheumatoid synovitis and pannus. In: Hochberg MC, Silman AJ, Smolen JS, Weinblatt ME, Weisman MH, editors. Rheumatology. 3rd ed. Philadelphia, USA: Mosby; 2003. pp. 855-884

[36] Schmidt D, Goronzy JJ, Weyand CM. CD4+ CD7− CD28− T cells are expanded in rheumatoid arthritis and are characterized by autoreactivity. The Journal of Clinical Investigation. 1996;**97**:2027-2037

[37] Ziff M. Role of endothelium in the pathogenesis of rheumatoid synovitis. International Journal of Tissue Reactions. 1993;**15**:135-137

[38] Roosnek E, Lanzavecchia A. Efficient and selective presentation of antigen-antibody complexes by rheumatoid factor B cells. The Journal of Experimental Medicine. 1991; **173**:487-489

[39] Sebbag M, Chapuy-Regaud S, Auger I, et al. Clinical and pathophysiological significance of the autoimmune response to citrullinated proteins in rheumatoid arthritis. Joint, Bone, Spine. 2004;**71**(6):493-502

[40] Young BJ, Mallya RK, Leslie RD. Anti-keratin antibodies in rheumatoid arthritis. British Medical Journal. 1979;**2**(6182):97-99

[41] Sokolove J, Bromberg R, Deane KD, et al. Autoantibody epitope spreading in the preclinical phase predicts progression to rheumatoid arthritis. PLoS One. 2012;**7**:5

[42] Goeb V, Jouen F, Gilbert D, Le Loet X, Tron F, Vittecoq O. Diagnostic and prognostic usefulness of antibodies to citrullinated peptides. Joint, Bone, Spine. 2009;**76**(4):343-349

[43] Alenius GM. Psoriatic arthritis-new insights give new options for treatment. Current Medicinal Chemistry. 2007;**14**(3):359-366

[44] Hendler A, Mulli TK, Hughes FJ, et al. Involvement of autoimmunity in the pathogenesis of aggressive periodontitis. Journal of Dental Research. 2010;**89**:1389-1394

[45] Strollo R, Ponchel F, Malmstrom V, et al. Autoantibodies to posttranslationally modified type II collagen as potential biomarkers for rheumatoid arthritis. Arthritis and Rheumatism. 2013;**65**(7):1702-1712

[46] Cruyssen BV, Cantaert T, Nogueira L, et al. Diagnostic value of anti-human citrullinated fibrinogen ELISA and comparison with four other anti-citrullinated protein assays. Arthritis Research & Therapy. 2006;**8**(4):R122

[47] Chapuy-Regaud S, Nogueira L, Clavel C, Sebbag M, Vincent C, Serre G. IgG subclass distribution of the rheumatoid arthritis-specific autoantibodies to citrullinated fibrin. Clinical & Experimental Immunology. 2005;**139**(3):542-550

[48] Masson-Bessi'ere C, Sebbag M, Girbal-Neuhauser E, et al. The major synovial targets of the rheumatoid arthritis-specific antifilaggrin autoantibodies are deiminated forms of the α-and β-chains of fibrin. The Journal of Immunology. 2001;**166**(6):4177-4184

[49] Sebbag M, Moinard N, Auger I, et al. Epitopes of human fibrin recognized by the rheumatoid arthritis-specific autoantibodies to citrullinated proteins. European Journal of Immunology. 2006;**36**(8):2250-2263

[50] Verpoort KN, Jol-van der Zijde CM, Papendrecht-van der Voort EA, et al. Isotype distribution of anti-cyclic citrullinated peptide antibodies in undifferentiated arthritis and rheumatoid arthritis reflects an ongoing immune response. Arthritis and Rheumatism. 2006;**54**(12):3799-3808

[51] van Beers JJ, Schwarte CM, Stammen-Vogelzangs J, et al. The rheumatoid arthritis synovial fluid citrullinome reveals novel citrullinated epitopes in apolipoprotein E, myeloid nuclear differentiation antigen, and beta-actin. Arthritis and Rheumatism. 2013;**65**(1):69-80

[52] Kuhn KA, Kulik L, Tomooka B, et al. Antibodies against citrullinated proteins enhance tissue injury in experimental autoimmune arthritis. The Journal of Clinical Investigation. 2006;**116**(4):961-973

[53] Scherer HU, van, der Woude D, Ioan-Facsinay A, et al. Glycan profiling of anti-citrullinated protein antibodies isolated from human serum and synovial fluid. Arthritis and Rheumatism. 2010;**62**(6):1620-1629

[54] Harre U, Lang SC, Pfeifle R, et al. Glycosylation of immunoglobulin G determines osteoclast differentiation and bone loss. Nature Communications. 2015;**6**:6651

[55] Kelley WN. Textbook of Rheumatology. 5th ed. Philadelphia: W.B. Saunders; 1997. pp. 626-685

[56] Kuettner KE, Aydelotte MB, Thonar EJ. Articular cartilage matrix and structure: A mini-review. The Journal of Rheumatology. Supplement. 1991;**27**:46-48

[57] Dodge GR, Pidoux I, Poole AR. The degradation of type II collagen in rheumatoid arthritis: An immunoelectron microscopic study. Matrix. 1991;**11**:330-338

[58] Morgan K. What do anti-collagen antibodies mean? Annals of the Rheumatic Diseases. 1990;**49**:62-65

[59] Kim WU, Yoo WH, Park W, Kang YM, Kim SI, Park JH, et al. IgG antibodies to type II collagen reflect inflammatory activity in patients with rheumatoid arthritis. The Journal of Rheumatology. 2000;**27**:575-581

[60] Mullazehi M, Mathsson L, Lampa J, Ronnelid J. High anti-collagen type-II antibody levels and induction of proinflammatory cytokines by anti-collagen antibody-containing immune complexes in vitro characterise a distinct rheumatoid arthritis phenotype associated with acute inflammation at the time of disease onset. Annals of the Rheumatic Diseases. 2007;**66**:537-541

[61] Lindh I, Snir O, Lönnblom E, Uysal H, Andersson I, Nandakumar KS, et al. Type II collagen antibody response is enriched in the synovial fluid of rheumatoid joints and directed to the same major epitopes as in collagen induced arthritis in primates and mice. Arthritis Research & Therapy. 2014;**16**:R143

[62] Morgan K, Clague RB, Collins I, Ayad S, Phinn SD, Holt PJ. Incidence of antibodies to native and denatured cartilage collagens (types II, IX, and XI) and to type I collagen in rheumatoid arthritis. Annals of the Rheumatic Diseases. 1987;**46**:902-907

[63] Mullazehi M, Mathsson L, Lampa J, Ronnelid J. Surface-bound anti-type II collagen-containing immune complexes induce production of tumor necrosis factor alpha, interleukin-1beta, and interleukin-8 from peripheral blood monocytes via Fc gamma receptor IIA: A potential pathophysiologic mechanism for humoral anti-type II collagen immunity in arthritis. Arthritis and Rheumatism. 2006;**54**:1759-1771

[64] Courtenay JS, Dallman MJ, Dayan AD, Martin A, Mosedale B. Immunisation against heterologous type II collagen induces arthritis in mice. Nature. 1980;**283**:666-668

[65] Wooley PH, Luthra HS, Stuart JM, David CS. Type II collagen-induced arthritis in mice. I. Major histocompatibility complex (I region) linkage and antibody correlates. The Journal of Experimental Medicine. 1981;**154**:688-700

[66] Svensson L, Jirholt J, Holmdahl R, Jansson L. B cell-deficient mice do not develop type II collagen-induced arthritis (CIA). Clinical and Experimental Immunology. 1998;**111**:521-526

[67] Wang Y, Kristan J, Hao L, Lenkoski CS, Shen Y, Matis LA. A role for complement in antibody-mediated inflammation: C5-deficient DBA/1 mice are resistant to collagen-induced arthritis. Journal of Immunology. 2000;**164**:4340-4347

[68] Burkhardt H, Koller T, Engström A, Nandakumar KS, Turnay J, Kraetsch HG, et al. Epitope-specific recognition of type II collagen by rheumatoid arthritis antibodies is shared with recognition by antibodies that are arthritogenic in collagen-induced arthritis in the mouse. Arthritis and Rheumatism. 2002;**46**:2339-2348

[69] Kraetsch HG, Unger C, Wernhoff P, Schneider C, Kalden JR, Holmdahl R, et al. Cartilage-specific autoimmunity in rheumatoid arthritis: Characterization of a triple helical B cell epitope in the integrin-binding-domain of collagen type II. European Journal of Immunology. 2001;**31**:1666-1673

[70] Nandakumar KS, Bajtner E, Hill L, Böhm B, Rowley MJ, Burkhardt H, et al. Arthritogenic antibodies specific for a major type II collagen triple-helical epitope bind and destabilize cartilage independent of inflammation. Arthritis and Rheumatism. 2008;**58**:184-196

[71] Nandakumar KS, Svensson L, Holmdahl R. Collagen type II-specific monoclonal antibody-induced arthritis in mice: Description of the disease and the influence of age, sex, and genes. The American Journal of Pathology. 2003;**163**:1827-1837

[72] Cook AD, Rowley MJ, Mackay IR, Gough A, Emery P. Antibodies to type II collagen in early rheumatoid arthritis. Correlation with disease progression. Arthritis and Rheumatism. 1996;**39**:1720-1727

[73] Burkhardt H, Sehnert B, Bockermann R, Engström A, Kalden JR, Holmdahl R. Humoral immune response to citrullinated collagen type II determinants in early rheumatoid arthritis. European Journal of Immunology. 2005;**35**:1643-1652

[74] Uysal H, Nandakumar KS, Kessel C, Haag S, Carlsen S, Burkhardt H, et al. Antibodies to citrullinated proteins: Molecular interactions and arthritogenicity. Immunological Reviews. 2010;**233**:9-33

[75] Brennan FM, McInnes IB. Evidence that cytokines play a role in rheumatoid arthritis. The Journal of Clinical Investigation. 2008;**118**(11):3537-3545

[76] Dayer JM, Beutler B, Cerami A. Cachectin/tumor necrosis factor stimulates collagenase and prostaglandin E2 production by human synovial cells and dermal fibroblasts. The Journal of Experimental Medicine. 1985;**162**:2163-2168

[77] Bertolini DR, Nedwin GE, Bringman TS, Smith DD, Mundy GR. Stimulation of bone resorption and inhibition of bone formation in vitro by human tumour necrosis factors. Nature. 1986;**319**:516-518

[78] Buchan G et al. Detection of activated T cell products in the rheumatoid joint using cDNA probes to Interleukin-2 (IL-2) IL-2 receptor and IFN-gamma. Clinical and Experimental Immunology. 1988;**71**:295-301

[79] Hirano T et al. Excessive production of interleukin 6/B cell stimulatory factor-2 in rheumatoid arthritis. European Journal of Immunology. 1988;**18**:1797-1801

[80] Haworth C et al. Expression of granulocytemacrophage colony-stimulating factor in rheumatoid arthritis: Regulation by tumor necrosis factoralpha. European Journal of Immunology. 1991;**21**:2575-2579

[81] Brennan FM et al. Detection of interleukin 8 biological activity in synovial fluids from patients with rheumatoid arthritis and production of interleukin 8 mRNA by isolated synovial cells. European Journal of Immunology. 1990;**20**:2141-2144

[82] Brennan FM, Chantry D, Jackson A, Maini R, Feldmann M. Inhibitory effect of TNF alpha antibodies on synovial cell interleukin-1 production in rheumatoid arthritis. Lancet. 1989;**2**:244-247

[83] Brennan FM, Chantry D, Jackson AM, Maini RN, Feldmann M. Cytokine production in culture by cells isolated from the synovial membrane. Journal of Autoimmunity. 1989;**2**(Suppl):177-186

[84] Kavanaugh AF, Schulze-Koops H, Davis LS, Lipsky PE. Repeat treatment of rheumatoid arthritis patients with a murine anti-intercellular adhesion molecule 1 monoclonal antibody. Arthritis and Rheumatism. 1997;**40**:849-853

[85] Deon D, Ahmed S, Tai K, et al. Cross-talk between IL-1 and IL-6 signaling pathways in rheumatoid arthritis synovial fibroblasts. Journal of Immunology. 2001;**167**:5395-5403

[86] Elliott MJ et al. Treatment of rheumatoid arthritis with chimeric monoclonal antibodies to tumor necrosis factor alpha. Arthritis and Rheumatism. 1993;**36**:1681-1690

[87] Elliott MJ et al. Randomised double-blind comparison of chimeric monoclonal antibody to tumour necrosis factor alpha (cA2) versus placebo in rheumatoid arthritis. Lancet. 1994;**344**:1105-1110

[88] Maini RN et al. Randomized placebo controlled trial of multiple intravenous infusions of anti-TNFα monoclonal antibody with or without weekly methotrexate in rheumatoid arthritis. Arthritis and Rheumatism. 1998;**41**:1552-1563

[89] Lipsky PE et al. 102 week clinical and radiological results from the ATTRACT trial: A 2 year, randomized, controlled, phase 3 trial of infliximab (Remicade) in patients with active rheumatoid arthritis despite methotrexate. Arthritis and Rheumatism. 2000;**47**(Suppl):S242

[90] Feldmann M, Maini RN. Anti-TNFα therapy or rheumatoid arthritis: What have we learned? Annual Review of Immunology. 2001;**19**:163-196

[91] Kay J, Calabrese L. The role of interleukin-1 in the pathogenesis of rheumatoid arthritis. Rheumatology. 2004;**43**(Suppl. 3):iii2-iii9

[92] Chomarat P, Vannier E, Dechanet J, et al. Balance of IL-1 receptor antagonist/IL-1 in rheumatoid synovium and its regulation by IL-4 and IL-10. Journal of Immunology. 1995;**154**:1432-1439

[93] Fontana A, Hengartner H, Weber E, Fehr K, Grob PJ, Cohen G. Interleukin 1 activity in the synovial fluid of patients with rheumatoid arthritis. Rheumatology International. 1982;**2**:49-53

[94] Weckmann AN, Alcocer-Varela J. Cytokine inhibitors in autoimmune disease. Seminars in Arthritis and Rheumatism. 1996;**26**:539-557

[95] Akira S, Taga T, Kishimoto T. Interleukin-6 in biology and medicine. Advances in Immunology. 1993;**54**:1-78

[96] Kishimoto T. Interleukin-6: From basic science to medicine-40 years in immunology. Annual Review of Immunology. 2005;**23**:1-21

[97] Muraguchi A, Hirano T, Tang B, Matsuda T, Horii Y, Nakajima K, et al. The essential role of B cell stimulatory factor 2 (BSF-2/IL-6) for the terminal differentiation of B cells. The Journal of Experimental Medicine. 1988;**167**:332-344

[98] Jogo G, Bataille R, Pellat-Deceunynck C. Interleukin-6 is a growth factor for nonmalignant human plasmablasts. Blood. 2001;**97**:1817-1822

[99] Dienz O, Eaton SM, Bond JP, Neveu W, Moquin D, Noubade R, et al. The induction of antibody production by IL-6 is indirectly mediated by IL-21 produced by CD4 T cells. The Journal of Experimental Medicine. 2009;**206**:69-78

[100] Dayer JM, Choy E. Therapeutic targets in rheumatoid arthritis: The interleukin-6 receptor. Rheumatology. 2010;**49**:15-24

[101] Lally F, Smith E, Filer A, et al. A novel mechanism of neutrophil recruitment in a coculture model of the rheumatoid synovium. Arthritis and Rheumatism. 2005;**52**:3460-3469

[102] Teitelbaum SL. Bone resorption by osteoclasts. Science. 2000;**289**:1504-1508

[103] Schett G. Cells of the synovium in rheumatoid arthritis. Osteoclasts. Arthritis Research & Therapy. 2007;**9**:203

[104] Paleolog EM. Angiogenesis in rheumatoid arthritis. Arthritis Research. 2002;**4**:S81-S90

[105] Keck PJ, Hauser SD, Krivi G, Sanzo K, Warren T, Feder J, et al. Vascular permeability factor, an endothelial cell mitogen related to PDGF. Science. 1989;**246**:1309-1312

[106] Ballara S, Taylor PC, Reusch P, Malme D, Feldmann M, Maini RN, et al. Raised serum vascular endothelial growth factor levels are associated with destructive change in inflammatory arthritis. Arthritis and Rheumatism. 2001;**44**:20552064

[107] Nakahara H, Song J, Sugimoto M, Hagihara K, Kishimoto T, Yoshizaki K, et al. Anti-interleukin-6 receptor antibody therapy reduces vascular endothelial growth factor production in rheumatoid arthritis. Arthritis and Rheumatism. 2003;**48**:1521-1529

[108] Choy EH, Isenberg DA, Garrood T, Farrow S, Ioannou Y, Bird H, et al. Therapeutic benefit of blocking interleukin-6 activity with an anti-interleukin-6 receptor monoclonal antibody in rheumatoid arthritis: A randomized, double-blind, placebo-controlled, dose-escalation trial. Arthritis and Rheumatism. 2002;**46**:3143-3150

[109] Nishimoto N, Yoshizaki K, Miyasaka N, Yamamoto K, Kawai K, Takeuchi T, et al. Treatment of rheumatoid arthritis with humanized anti-interleukin-6 receptor antibody: A multicenter, double-blind, placebo-controlled trial. Arthritis and Rheumatism. 2004;**50**:1761-1769

[110] Maini RN, Taylor PC, Szechinski J, Pavelka K, Broll J, Balint G, et al. Double-blind randomized controlled clinical trial of the interleukin-6 receptor antagonist, tocilizumab, in European patients with rheumatoid arthritis who had an incomplete response to methotrexate. Arthritis and Rheumatism. 2006;**54**:2817-2829

[111] Smolen JS, Beaulieu A, Rubbert-Roth A, Ramos-Remus C, Rovensky J, Alecock E, et al. Effect of interleukin-6 receptor inhibition with tocilizumab in patients with rheumatoid arthritis (OPTION study): A double-blind, placebo-controlled, randomised trial. Lancet. 2008;**371**:987-997

[112] Genovese MC, McKay JD, Nasonov EL, Mysler EF, da Silva NA, Alecock E, et al. Interleukin-6 receptor inhibition with tocilizumab reduces disease activity in rheumatoid arthritis with inadequate response to disease-modifying antirheumatic drugs: The tocilizumab in combination with traditional disease-modifying antirheumatic drug therapy study. Arthritis and Rheumatism. 2008;**58**:2968-2980

[113] Emery P, Keystone E, Tony HP, Cantagrel A, van Vollenhoven R, Sanchez A, et al. IL-6 receptor inhibition with tocilizumab improves treatment outcomes in patients with rheumatoid arthritis refractory to anti-tumour necrosis factor biologicals: Results from a 24-week multicentre randomised placebo-controlled trial. Annals of the Rheumatic Diseases. 2008;**67**:1516-1523

[114] Nishimoto N, Hashimoto J, Miyasaka N, Yamamoto K, Kawai S, Takeuchi T, et al. Study of active controlled monotherapy used for rheumatoid arthritis, an IL-6 inhibitor (SAMURAI): Evidence of clinical and radiographic benefit from an x ray reader-blinded randomised controlled trial of tocilizumab. Annals of the Rheumatic Diseases. 2007;**66**:1162-1167

[115] Fleischmann R, Burgos-Vargas R, Ambs P, Alecock E, Kremer J. LITHE: Tocilizumab inhibits radiographic progression and improves physical function in rheumatoid arthritis (RA) patients (Pts) at 2 Yrs with increasing clinical efficacy over time. Arthritis and Rheumatism. 2009;**60**(10):S238-S239

[116] Caporali R, Idolazzi L, Bombardieri S. Tocilizumab in the treatment of patients with rheumatoid arthritis in real clinical practice: Results of an Italian observational study. Clinical and Experimental Rheumatology. 2017;**35**(6):919-928

[117] Rubbert-Roth A, Furst DE, Nebesky JM, Jin A, Berber E. A review of recent advances using tocilizumab in the treatment of rheumatic diseases. Rheumatology and Therapy. 2018;**5**(1):21-24

Chapter 7

Primary Sjögren's Syndrome and Autoantibodies

Maria Maślińska and Brygida Kwiatkowska

Additional information is available at the end of the chapter

http://dx.doi.org/10.5772/intechopen.75011

Abstract

The presence of certain autoantibodies in the serum of patients facilitates the diagnosis of particular autoimmune diseases. Some antibodies may also be significant for the prognosis of the disease development and internal organs involvement. In the case of Sjögren's syndrome, it is known that overactivity of B-lymphocytes leads to the production of a number of autoantibodies—both markers for pSS (such as antibodies to ribonucleoproteins) and nonspecific antibodies (such as rheumatoid factor). The range of autoantibodies found in pSS is constantly expanding, but their significance is not fully established. At present, only anti-SS-A antibodies are introduced to the criteria for the pSS diagnosis. However, this does not stop an interest in other autoantibodies and the significance of their presence for the course of this disease. This chapter outlines the autoantibodies found in pSS and discusses their importance in clinical practice.

Keywords: primary Sjögren's syndrome, autoantibodies, clinical association

1. Introduction

Primary Sjögren's syndrome (pSS) is a chronic, persistent autoimmune disease with predominant B cells hyperreactivity and with the production of autoantibodies against intracellular antigens. Autoimmune process taking place in pSS affects exocrine glands primarily, causing their dysfunction and the development of symptoms of mouth and eye dryness. Through the formation of infiltrates consisting of different autoreactive cells (e.g., B and T cells, macrophages, and dendritic cells), pSS may affect other organs as well as whole systems (e.g., lungs, respiratory, urinary, and alimentary tract).

1.1. Triggering factors

In the pathogenesis of primary Sjögren's syndrome, certain genetic factors play a significant role, such as the presence of HLA-B8, HLA-DW3, HLA-DR3, and DRw52 genes or interferon regulatory factor 5 (IRF 5) gene polymorphism [1, 2]. Not only viral infections have been recognized as the pSS triggering factors, mainly Epstein-Barr virus (EBV) [3], but also human T-cell lymphotropic virus type-1 (HTLV-1), cytomegalovirus (CMV), and hepatitis C virus (HCV) [4, 5]. Bacterial infections *Staphylococcus aureus, Chlamydia pneumoniae, Chlamydia trachomatis, M. hominis, U. urealyticum*, and *H. pylori* may also play part in the development of pSS [6–8]. In many of the autoimmune rheumatic diseases, ultraviolet (UV) radiation is a recognized factor influencing the activity of the autoimmune process. The UV radiation causes movement of antigen molecules, bound with/to ribonucleoprotein, between cytoplasm and cell membrane (SS-A/Ro) and cell nucleus and cytoplasm (SS-B/La). UVB radiation affects epithelial damage, activates plasma dendritic cells, and increases the risk of their apoptosis and (risk?) of the IFN signaling pathway activation. Different observations concerning UVA radiation suggest that it inhibits the production of autoantibodies [9, 10].

The hormonal state of the individual may also play a role in the pSS development. The imbalance of sex hormones and its receptors, dependent on hypothalamic-pituitary-adrenal axis (HPA or HTPA axis), interferes with the ratio of estrogens to androgens, especially in genetically predisposed patients [11]. This influences the stimulation of the autoimmune process and may explain the more frequent occurrence of pSS in women, especially in middle-aged. In recent years, attention has been paid to the role of the deficiency of dehydroepiandrosterone (DHEA) and of DHEA-S, its metabolite, in pSS and other autoimmune diseases [12].

1.2. Outline of pathogenesis

As the epithelial cell damage and apoptosis provide basis for the pSS pathogenesis, the first step of the whole process is the activation of innate immunity, as the virus or bacteria antigen activates pattern recognition receptors (PRR) via Toll-like receptors (especially TLR 3, 7, 9). Activation of innate immunity leads, in turn, to the damage of epithelial cells, their apoptosis and the release of antigens and RNA complexes that strongly stimulate plasmacytoid dendritic cells (pDCs). These produce interferon alpha (IFN-α)—a factor strongly stimulating epithelial cells, dendritic cells and neutrophils to produce B-cell activating factor (BAFF) [13–16]. All processes initiating epithelial damage lead to the apoptosis of cells, activation of congenital and acquired immune systems and the cascade effect of pathophysiological phenomena, resulting primarily in the overproduction of BAFF and other B-cell stimulating cytokines including APRIL (proliferation inducing ligand), similar in its actions to BAFF. Both BAFF and APRIL belong to the tumor necrosis factor superfamily (TNF) [17, 18]. The antigens released from damaged cells, primarily SS-A and SS-B ribonucleoproteins are targets for B cells and cause the production of specific anti-SS-A/Ro and anti-SS-B/La autoantibodies. Plasmocytoid dendritic cells also stimulate T lymphocytes, particularly the CD4+ subtype, which is later the main component of infiltrates in the endocrine glands. The Th1-type immune response is predominant, with activation of Th17 cells secreting interleukin 17 (IL-17). Th1 cells produce IFN-γ, which, in addition to the increase of BAFF secretion, induces the production of plasminogen activator, which—simultaneously with IL-17—causes the development of local inflammatory process. As a result of the abovementioned changes, leading to the hyperstimulation of B lymphocytes, autotolerance is disturbed and further production of autoantibodies [19].

2. Autoantibodies in primary Sjögren's syndrome

2.1. Antinuclear antibodies

A primary test for autoantibodies, finding the use in the diagnostics of pSS and other systemic autoimmune rheumatic diseases (SARD), is the determination of anti-nuclear antibodies (ANAs) [20, 21]. ANA are found in 80–90% of patients with pSS. These antibodies react with the components of the cell nucleus and are most often tested with indirect immunofluorescence (IF) on HEp-2 (human epithelial cell) cell line. In pSS, ANA often occur in higher titers (above 1:320), but may be also detected in lower titers (1:160) and in the concurrent presence of other autoantibodies. In **Table 1**, the prevalence of ANA antibodies in different autoimmune diseases was presented.

In recent years attention has been paid to the frequent occurrence of dense fine speckled pattern (DFS70) on HEp-2 in both healthy people and patients with ANA associated autoimmune rheumatic diseases (AARD). DFS70 antibodies bind a ubiquitinated protein called lens epithelium derived growth factor (LEDGF), which occurrence was associated in first observations [22] with asthma and atopic dermatitis. However, the high prevalence of DFS70 autoantibodies in normal population, without any symptoms of any AARD, was observed. Therefore, in the case of positive result of the screening for ANA antibodies in individuals without symptoms suggestive of a systemic autoimmune rheumatic disease (SARD/AARD), it is advisable to detect DFS70 antibodies using specific tests (e.g., ELISA/EIA; CLIA/CIA) [23, 24]. Even up to 1/3 of positive cases for ANA are also positive for DFS70 antibodies [23, 24].

2.2. Extractable nuclear antigens

In 1959, Holman et al. recorded a reaction of sera from SLE patients with extractable nuclear antigens (ENA) isolated from a crushed calf thymus. This observation confirmed the reaction of autoantibodies in the SLE sera with soluble nuclear antigens. The nomenclature of ENA autoantibodies derived from the group, in which they were first described, and corresponds to the nuclear function of the antigen (RNP) or the name of the patient providing the prototype serum (Ro, La, Sm, Jo, Mi), as well as the disease from which the patient suffered (SSA,

Disease	SLE	SSc	pSS	MCTD
ANA sensitivity%	95	70–90	50–80	90

SLE—systemic lupus erythematosus; SS, SSc—systemic sclerosis, pSS—primary Sjögren's syndrome, MCTD—mixed connective tissue disease.

Table 1. Prevalence of ANA antibodies in different autoimmune diseases [20, 21].

SSB, SSC, Scl-70, PM-1, PM-Scl) [23]. The set of all ENA includes more than 100 soluble and cytoplasmic antigens. In clinical practice, until present day, only few of the them are finding use as a immunological hallmarks of certain autoimmune diseases or being used as immunological prognostic factors. Among them the most prominent are as follows: anti-RNP (anti-ribonucleoprotein anti-U(1)RNP), anti-Sm RNP, anti-SSA/Ro, anti-SSB/La, anti-Sm (Smith) antibody, anti-Scl-70 (anti-topoisomerase antibodies), anti-Jo-1 (anti-histidyl-transfer RNA synthase antibodies). The pattern of positive and negative results obtained with an ENA panel should be evaluated in conjunction with all clinical findings. Main autoantibodies and disease which they are typical to are presented in **Table 2**. Selected autoimmune diseases along with their predominant autoantibodies are presented in **Table 2. Figure 1** shows a simplified diagnostic algorithm of immunological diagnosis.

2.3. Characteristics of ENA antibodies and their connection with primary Sjögren's syndrome

From 1981, it is known [26] that SS-A/Ro antigens are associated with small cytoplasmic RNAs. In 1984 Ro60 kD protein was discovered and Ben-Chetrit et al. in 1988 demonstrated second part of SS-A/Ro complex—a 52 kD protein [25–27]. As we have recently learned, the SS-A/Ro antigen consists of two different proteins Ro60 and Ro 52, with different gene localization: Ro60 is located on chromosome 19, while Ro-52 on chromosome 11. It was also revealed that these antigens, in physiological conditions, are found in different cell compartments. The detection of their presence determines different clinical implications. Presently, this problem needs still further investigation.

SS-A/Ro (60KD + 52KD) is a complex present on most cells, including platelets and red blood cells. It is considered that the anti-SS-A antibody plays a pathogenic role in pSS and its presence is associated with more severe symptoms, resulting from the involvement of endocrine glands, lymphadenopathy, larger salivary glandular infiltrates, characteristic vasculitis and longer duration of the disease [28, 29]. Also the occurrence of interstitial lung disease (ILD) is

Disease.	RA	pSS	MCTD	SLE	dSSc	lSSc	PM	DM	GPA	MPA
Antibodies	ACPA RF	Anti-SS-A/Ro60 Anti-SS-A/Ro52 Anti-SS-B/LA RF	RNP RF	Anti-dsDNA Anti-Sm Anti-Ro60	Anti-Scl-70	Anti-CENP-A,B,C	Anti-Jo-1 Ro-52 Other anti-synthetase antibodies, Anti-Mi-2 Anti-SRP	Anti-Ro-52 Anti-Mi-2	cANCA	pANCA

RA—rheumatoid arthritis; pSS—primary Sjogren's syndrome; MCTD—mixed connective tissue disese; SLE—systemic lupus erythematosus; dSSc—disseminated systemic sclerosis, lSSc-localized systemic sclerosis; PM—polymyositis; DM—dermatomyosistis; GPA—granulomatosis with polyangiitis; MPA—microscopic polyangiitis.

Table 2. Autoimmune diseases and main autoantibodies [20–24].

http://dx.doi.org/10.5772/intechopen.75011

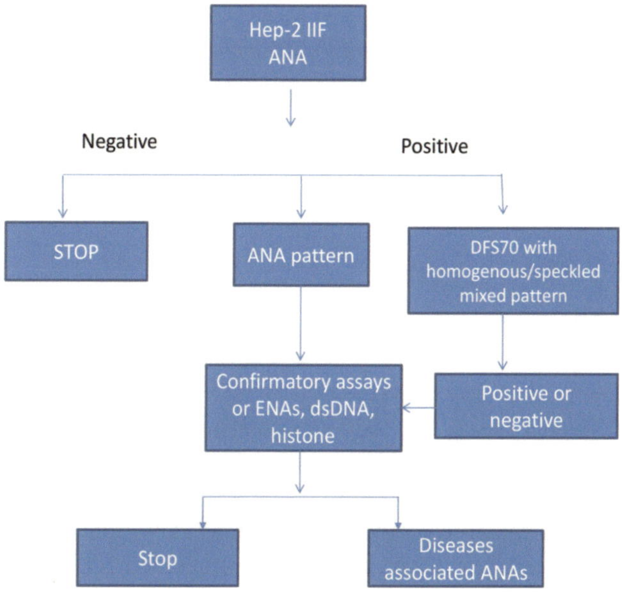

Figure 1. Simplified algorithm of immunological diagnosis of rheumatic diseases [22–24]. ANA—antinuclear antibodies; DFS70—dense fine speckled pattern antibodies; ENAs—extractable nuclear antigens; dsDNA—anti-double stranded DNA antibodies.

associated with the presence of antibodies against SS-A/Ro antigens, primarily Ro52KD and is associated with a higher degree of inflammatory changes in the salivary glands.

The formation of anti-SS-A is affected by the UV radiation, which increases the expression of antigens on the cell surface. Anti-SS-A/Ro antibodies are considered as a triggering factor for photosensitivity in SCLE and NLE, although patients with DLE, but without anti-Ro antibodies, present skin changes after sun/light exposition as well, probably due to other pathomechanism (the presence of autoantibodies/immunoglobulins between skin and the epidermis) [30].

Ro60 antigen attaches to uncoded RNA to form a complex (hY-RNA) that plays a role in inhibiting the immune response. Ro52 antigen is a phosphoprotein forming due to stimulation by viral infection, type I interferon pathway and through Toll-like receptors [28].

2.3.1. Anti-SSA/Ro antibodies

Autoantibody Ro60 has been associated with Sjögren's syndrome in particular but also occur in SLE (50%), and subacute cutaneous lupus (SCLE) (60%) and neonatal lupus (NLE) [31]. Anti-Ro antibodies in SLE and SCLE are associated with photosensivity and skin changes (SCLE, NLE). In SCLE, negative results for ANA screening or finding ANA in low titer do not exclude the presence of anti-SSA/Ro antibodies (antibody—negative SCLE). Anti-SS-A antibodies are also found in systemic sclerosis, RA and polymyositis, as well as dermatomyositis (PM/DM) and autoimmune hepatitis, with antibodies to the Ro52 antigen present more frequently. Anti-Ro52 antibodies frequently occur in association with anti-Ro60 antibodies, especially in the context of SLE, Sjögren's syndrome, subacute cutaneous lupus and neonatal lupus congenital heart block [31, 32]. However, the presence of anti-Ro52 alone, without anti-Ro60, was reported in inflammatory myopathy and in systemic sclerosis. It was also observed, that anti-Ro52 antibodies are, to larger extent than anti-Ro60, associated with primary biliary cirrhosis (PBC) and autoimmune hepatitis (AIH) with co-expression of anti SLA antibodies (soluble liver antibodies) [33].

2.3.2. Anti-SS-B/La antibodies

Anti-SS-B/La antibodies are less common and usually coexist with anti-SS-A antibodies, and their presence in other systemic diseases, especially in SLE (25% of patients with TRU), is associated with skin lesions (erythema, alopecia), inflammation of the serous membranes, leukopenia, symptoms of dryness and they often coexist with the presence of anti-SS-A antibodies (secondary SS) [28]. Rao et al. have noted that anti-SSB antibodies are important for the SLE diagnosis. They are associated with cheek erythema, alopecia, serositis, secondary Sjögren's syndrome, and hematological changes such as leukocytopenia, thrombocytopenia, and immunoglobulins elevation. They are often accompanied by the presence of anti-/Ro or anti-SSA/Ro52 antibodies [34]. These autoantibodies may also be found before the SLE-specific antibodies can be detected [35].

3. Rheumatoid factor

Rheumatoid factor (RF) is an autoantibody directed against the CH2 and CH3 domains of an Fc region of a class G immunoglobulin (IgG). RF is produced by plasmatic cells (RF-PCs) that are formed from B cells activated both dependently and independently of T lymphocytes. Thus, RF producing B cells (RF-PC) become cells with ability of antigen presentation (APC) and of binding IgG. As this cascade of events constitutes a method of immune response against the infectious antigens, the RF production during infections protects the host organism. This phenomenon explains the occurrence of RF in the course of many viral (e.g., HCV, Herpes virus, and HIV), bacterial (e.g., subacute bacterial endocarditis, *Chlamydia pneumoniae*, *Klebsiella pneumoniae*, tuberculosis, and syphilis) and even parasitic (malaria, onchocerciasis, and toxoplasmosis) infections. In those autoimmune diseases, in which B-cell hyperactivity occurs, rheumatoid factors, particularly clinically relevant RF-IgM, also appears [36]. It should be remembered that RF appears in 4% of a healthy population and its incidence increases with age; after 75 years of life, RF can be observed even in 10–25% of individuals [37, 38]. The frequency (%) of RF in various CTD is presented in **Table 3**. The primary Sjögren's syndrome is one of the autoimmune diseases in which the majority of patients have a rheumatoid factor (some authors report up from 60 to 90% of patients)—specifically its most common IgM class isotype. The presence of RF IgM is associated with the occurrence of leukopenia, increased erythrocyte sedimentation rate (ESR), higher concentration of gamma globulins and lower C4 complement component concentration. Observations of a positive correlation of the rheumatoid factor with symptoms of dryness, hypergammaglobulinemia, presence of higher ANA antibody titers, presence of

http://dx.doi.org/10.5772/intechopen.75011

Autoimmune connective tissue disease	RF frequency%
Primary Sjögren's syndrome	75–90
Rheumatoid arthritis	70–90
Mixed connective tissue disease	50–60
Systemic sclerosis	20–30
Systemic lupus erythematosus	15–20
Dermato/polymyositis	20
Vasculitis (GPA and MPA)	5–20
Other CTD* as psoriatic arthritis, juvenile idiopathic arthritis, and reactive arthritis	5 and <5

Table 3. The frequency of RF in various connective tissue diseases [39].

anti-SS-A antibodies, anti-SS-B, increased ESR and leukopenia were presented in their work by Witte et al. [39]. The presence of RF in patients with pSS, as well as in other autoimmune diseases, and in acute infections, indicates the formation of a large number of other antibodies and the formation of antigen complexes with antibodies. The frequency of RF in various CTD was presented in **Table 3** [39].

4. Other autoantibodies

4.1. Anti-centromere autoantibodies

Anti-centromere antibodies (ACA) are directed to six antigens associated with centromere (composed of a complex of kinetochore proteins). Currently identified anti-centromere antibodies (CENP) have been assigned designations with letters from A to F. The most common are CENP-A, B and C. CENP-B is also the most frequently occurring anti-centromere antibody in patients with pSS. The incidence of ACA antibody described in the literature ranges from 3.7 to 4% [40, 41]. This antibody, with a mass of 80 kDa, is a DNA-binding protein involved in the heterochromatin folding. Anti-centromere antibodies (A, B, C) occur mainly in limited systemic sclerosis (LSSc) and are associated with the prevalence of telangiectasia, higher severity of Raynaud's symptom, lung involvement such as interstitial lung disease [ILD] and fibrosis [42]. Their relationship between the presence of ACA antibodies and the involvement of endocrine glands has been demonstrated; in the ACA+ group, anti-SS-A and anti-SS-B autoantibodies were less frequent [42].

The association of ACA antibodies with non-Hodgkin's lymphomas (CENP-F) including MALT lymphomas was also described [43], as well as the case reports of CENP-B presence in small-cell lung cancer [44].

Interestingly, it has also been demonstrated that the presence of anti-CENP-B antibodies is associated with prolonged survival in a breast cancer [45].

4.2. Antibodies against citrullinated proteins

Citrullination is the post-translational process in proteins of deamination/conversion of the amino acids: arginine into citrulline. ACPA positive sera include antibodies to citrullinated proteins, such as fibrin and fibrinogen, vimentine (MCV—mutated citrullinated vimentine) and alpha-enolase (CEP-1).

It is known that arthritis may be one of the clinical symptoms of pSS. However, most of the pSS patients suffer from arthralgia, and only minority develop non-destructive arthritis. ACPA antibodies, a main marker of rheumatoid arthritis, are usually present in low concentrations in pSS according to various studies they are present in 3–22% of cases [46]. A higher incidence of arthritis was found in pSS patients with ACPA presence compared to patients without these antibodies [47]. It seems, however, that patients with pSS and ACPA positive require further observation toward the development of rheumatoid arthritis [48].

It should also be remembered that smoking and periodontal infection by *Porphyromonas gingivalis* are strong environmental factors stimulating protein citrullination and the emergence of ACPA antibodies [49].

4.3. Citrullinated alpha-enolase

Citrullinated alpha enolase (CEP-1) is an antigenic target for antibodies against citrullinated proteins (ACPA). In the Nezos et al. study [50], it was shown that CEP-1 antigen is a major antigen target in the ACPA positive subgroup of patients with pSS. The frequency of CEP-1 antibody in the RA ACPA positive group was not as high, while it was not found healthy group at all. The authors drew attention to the link of anti-CEP-1 antibodies presence to arthritis as well as to renal tubular dysfunction.

4.4. Antibodies recognizing salivary gland and lacrimal gland tissue

In recent years, researchers identified autoantibodies to carbonic anhydrase 6 (anti-CA6 antibodies), anti salivary gland protein 1 (SP-1) and anti-parotid secretory protein (PSP) [51]. These antibodies may emerge before pSS marker antibodies such as SS-A/Ro or SS-B/La and are associated with a minor focus score; these antibodies also occur more often in patients who did not have anti-SS-A/Ro antibodies [52]. Interestingly, in Langhe et al. work, anti CA6-IgA antibodies were detected primarily in patients with long pSS duration; other autoantibodies such as anti-CA6, PSP, and SP1 in IgG and IgM class were more frequently observed in SSc and MCTD with secondary SS. These autoantibodies do not allow distinguishing SLE from secondary SS. However, the described study was limited by a small group of SLE patients [52]. In the literature, some cases have been reported of patients with severe symptoms of eye or mouth dryness, in which there was no SS-A/Ro antibodies, but the presence of anti SP-1 antibody was confirmed [53]. It may suggest, that in case of a patients presenting unexplained dryness with no serology markers defined in current criteria for pSS, performing the test for novel, early antibodies to Sp1 and PSP may still be useful for diagnosing patient's condition [53].

4.5. Anti-muscarinic antibodies

Muscarinic 3 receptor (M3R) is found in various places in the body, such as smooth muscles, the endocrine and the exocrine glands, lungs, pancreas and even the brain. This receptor is also expressed on pancreatic beta cells, modulating insulin secretion. Activation of the M3R receptor induces smooth muscle constriction and increase glandular secretions [54].

It has been demonstrated that muscarinic acetylcholine type 3 receptor (M3R) antibodies are present in the serum of patients with pSS [54]. As it was presented by Kovacs et al., M3R antibodies are found in up to 90% of subjects with pSS [55]. In the group with M3R antibodies, leucopenia was more frequently observed [55]. Immune response to muscarinic receptor 3 plays a role in the pathogenesis of autoimmune sialoadenitis [56] and diabetes mellitus type 2. MR3 antibodies may be present in other autoimmune diseases and do not allow for differentiation between primary and secondary Sjögren's syndrome. The severity of symptoms of dryness or dysfunction of the exocrine system in pSS may be related not only to MR3 antibodies presence but also to other autoantibodies such as, for example, antibodies to aquaporins [57].

4.6. Autoantibodies to aquaporins

Aquaporins (AQP; water channels) are integral membrane proteins that form pores in the membrane of biological cells, enabling transport of water between cells. Some genetic defects of aquaporin genes have been associated with diseases as neuromyelitis optica (Devic's syndrome) and nephrogenic diabetes insipidus. First, aquaporin—"aquaporin-1" was described in 1992 by Peter Agre, until today we know 13 aquaporins, of which four are best defined [58]. Because of their influence of water transport, aquaporins have an impact on saliva and tear production and changes in AQP expression may lead to dryness symptoms [59, 60]. Aquaporin-4 (AQP4) is found on perivascular and ependymal cells, but it has also been discovered in sera of patients with NMO and multiple sclerosis. Tzartos and his colleagues detected aquaporin antibodies (AQP-1, -3, -8, and -9) in pSS patients sera [61]. What is interesting in the pSS group, AQP-4 and AQP-5 antibodies were not present. The presence of AQP antibodies was associated with more severe xeropthalmia; the authors suggest potential role of AQ P-Ab in salivary gland secretions. Such hypothesis requires further research.

4.7. Autoantibodies binding to stathmin-4

Stathmins (STMN) are phosphoproteins which play a role in neuronal development and interact with tubulin. Presently, four stathmins have been identified. Stathmins are upregulated in a number of cancers and neuropathies [62]. Anti-stathmin-4 antibodies in IgG3 class were proposed as a biomarker of polyneuropathy and such observations were presented by Duda et al. in their study. The authors described anti-STMN4 antibodies in 33% of pSS patients with polyneuropathy (PNP)—vs. 7% of those without PNP—and in 45% of individuals with vasculitis skin changes (as opposed to 13% in individuals without them) [63].

4.8. Anti-alpha-fodrin antibodies

Alpha fodrin is an actin-binding, organ-specific protein of the cytoskeleton. Antibodies against alpha-fodrin are detected in serum samples from patients with primary or secondary Sjögren's syndrome especially with sicca symptoms. Some authors suggest that they can be detected earlier in the course of pSS, sometimes before the emergence of anti SS-A or SS-B antibodies [64]. These antibodies, in the IgA and IgG class of immunoglobulins, are found in the serum and salivary glands of patients with pSS. However, other researchers did not describe any significant sensitivity and specificity of these antibodies [65–67].

4.9. Autoantibodies in saliva that may be relevant in pSS associated with the development of MALT lymphoma

Major salivary glands are the main extra endocrine glands targeted in pSS and saliva of patients with pSS is also a source of antibodies and cytokines. Large salivary glands are also the site for MALT lymphoma development. Investigators are interested in finding biomarkers in saliva, that allow for early pSS diagnosis, as well as the detection of mucosa associated lymphoma (MALT lymphoma). Cui et al. suggest set of three autoantibodies such as anti-cofilin-1 antibodies, anti-alpha enolase and anti-Rho GDP dissociation inhibitor 2(RGI2) antibodies, which, due to high specificity and sensitivity, may play a role as such biomarkers [68].

5. Autoantibodies in course of pSS—summary

In the current pSS criteria, only anti-SS-A/Ro antibodies are taken into account as the most sensitive and specific for pSS diagnosis. Still, the multisymptom picture of this rheumatic disease compels the search for other immunologic markers of at least equal prognostic importance.

Auto-antibody	Clinical findings
Anti-Ro52 kD	Interstitial lung disease
Anti-Ro60 kD	Hematologic changes, photosensitivity, skin involvement, Raynaud's phenomena, and dryness
Anti-SS-B/La	Liver (autoimmune disease) PBC
RF	Dryness, hypergammaglobulinemia, and leukopenia
ACPA	Arthralgia and arthritis
Anti-CENP-B	Interstitial lung disease and fibrosis
Novel autoantibodies	
Anti-CA6	Dryness and renal tubular acidosis
Anti-PSP	Dryness
Anti-SP1	Dryness
Anti-CEP-1	Arthritis and renal tubular dysfunction.

Table 4. Antibodies in pSS and their association with clinical manifestation.

http://dx.doi.org/10.5772/intechopen.75011

The occurrence of some of the identified antibodies has been associated with the specific clinical features such as interstitial lung disease, increased eye dryness, increased risk of nephrolithiasis and tubular distal acidosis or MALT lymphomas. In **Table 4**, autoantibodies frequently occurring in pSS and their association with clinical manifestation were presented.

6. Conclusions

pSS is a still not fully understood autoimmune disease, requiring doctor's vigilance. Even despite of a pSS having a mild course for a long time, there is a risk of organs and systems involvement. As it has been known for many years already, the risk of developing lymphomas is particularly increased in pSS patients compared to the healthy population. Although only one antibody (SS-A/Ro) has been included in the pSS diagnostic criteria, a lot of attention has been paid to new autoantibodies that can help clinicians in patient stratification in the early stages of diagnosis or may have a prognostic value.

Conflict of interest

The authors declare no conflict of interest.

Author details

Maria Maślińska* and Brygida Kwiatkowska

*Address all correspondence to: maslinskam@gmail.com

Early Arthritis Clinic, National Institute of Geriatrics, Rheumatology and Rehabilitation, Warsaw, Poland

References

[1] Cruz-Tapias P, Rojas-Villarraga A, Maier-Moore S, Anaya JM. HLA and Sjögren's syndrome susceptibility. A meta-analysis of worldwide studies. Autoimmunity Reviews. 2012;**11**:281-287

[2] Ciccacci C, Perricone C, Ceccarelli F, et al. A multilocus genetic study in a cohort of Italian SLE patients confirms the association with STAT4 gene and describes a new association with HCP5 gene. PLoS One. 2014;**9**:e111991

[3] Crawford DH. Biology and disease associations of Epstein-Barr virus. Philosophical Transactions of the Royal Society of London. Series B, Biological Sciences. 2001;**356**:461-473

[4] Niller HH, Wolf H, Minarovits J. Regulation and dysregulation of Epstein-Barr virus latency: Implications for the development of autoimmune diseases. Autoimmunity. 2008;**41**:298-328

[5] Ramos-Casals M, Garcia-Carrasco M, Cervera R, Font J. Is hepatitis C virus a sialotropic virus? The American Journal of Pathology. 2001;**159**:1593-1594

[6] Igoe A, Scofield RH. Autoimmunity and infection in Sjogren's syndrome. Current Opinion in Rheumatology. 2013;**25**:480-487

[7] Smyk DS, Koutsoumpas AL, Mytilinaiou MG, et al. Helicobacter pylori and autoimmune disease: Cause or bystander. World Journal of Gastroenterology. 2014;**20**:613-629

[8] Theander E, Nilsson I, Manthorpe R, et al. Seroprevalence of helicobacter pylori in primary Sjögren's syndrome. Clinical and Experimental Rheumatology. 2001;**19**:633-638

[9] McGrath H Jr. Ultraviolet-A1 irradiation decreases clinical disease activity and autoantibodies in patients with systemic lupus erythematosus. Clinical and Experimental Rheumatology. 1994;**12**:129-135

[10] Yin Q, Xu X, Lin Y, et al. Ultraviolet B irradiation induces skin accumulation of plasmacytoid dendritic cells: A possible role for chemerin. Autoimmunity. 2014;**47**:185-192

[11] Tzioufas AG, Tsonis J, Moutsopoulos HM. Neuroendocrine dysfunction in Sjogren's syndrome. Neuroimmunomodulation. 2008;**15**:37-45

[12] Virkki LM, Porola P, Forsblad-d'Elia H, et al. Dehydroepiandrosterone (DHEA) substitution treatment for severe fatigue in DHEA-deficient patients with primary Sjögren's syndrome. Arthritis Care & Research (Hoboken). 2010;**62**:118-124

[13] Youinou P, Pers JO. Disturbance of cytokine networks in Sjögren's syndrome. Arthritis Research & Therapy. 2011;**13**:227

[14] Pers JO, Lahiri A, Tobón GJ, Youinou P. Pathophysiological cytokine network in primary Sjögren's syndrome. Presse Médicale. 2012;**41**:e467-e474

[15] Mackay F, Groom JR, Tangye SG. An important role for B-cell activation factor and B cells in the pathogenesis of Sjogren's syndrome. Current Opinion in Rheumatology. 2007;**19**:406-413

[16] Kroese FG, Abdulahad WH, Haacke E, et al. B-cell hyperactivity in primary Sjögren's syndrome. Expert Review of Clinical Immunology. 2014;**10**:483-499

[17] Kontny E, Maśliński W. Limfocyty B—funkcje fizjologiczne i udział w patogenezie reumatoidalnego zapalenia stawów. Reumatologia. 2006;**44**:150-161

[18] Daridon C, Youinou P, Pers JO. BAFF, APRIL, TWE-PRIL: Who's who? Autoimmunity Reviews. 2008;**7**:267-271

[19] Mackay F, Leung H. The role of the BAFF/APRIL system on T cell function. Seminars in Immunology. 2006;**18**:284289

[20] Soto ME, Hernández-Becerril N, Perez-Chiney AC, et al. Predictive value of antinuclear antibodies in autoimmune diseases classified by clinical criteria: Analytical study in a specialized health institute, one year follow-up. Results in Immunology. 2015;**5**:13-22. DOI: 10.1016/j.rinim.2013.10.003

[21] Kyriakidis NC, Kapsogeorgou EK, Tzioufas AGA. Comprehensive review of autoantibodies in primary Sjogren's syndrome: Clinical phenotypes and regulatory mechanisms. Journal of Autoimmunity. 2003;**51C**:67-74

[22] Ochs RL, Mahler M, Basu A, et al. The significance of autoantibodies to DSF70/LEDGFp75 in health and disease: Integrating basic science with clinical understanding. Clinical and Experimental Medicine. 2016;**16**:273-293

[23] Shovman O, Gilburd B, Chayat C, et al. Prevalence of anti-DFS70 antibodies in patients with and without systemic autoimmune rheumatic diseases. Clinical and Experimental Rheumatology. 2017 [Epub ahead of print]

[24] Malyavantham K, Suresh L. Analysis of DFS pattern and impact on ANA screening using a novel Hep-2 ELITE/DFS70 knockout substrate. Autoimmunity Highlights. 2017;**8**:3

[25] Wenzel J, Gerdsen R, Uerlich M, Bauer R, Bieber T, Boehm I. Antibodies targeting extractable nuclear antigens: Historical development and current knowledge. British Journal of Dermatology. 2002;**145**(6):859-867

[26] Lerner MR, Boyle JA, Hardin JA, Steitz JA. Two novel classes of small ribonucleoproteins detected by antibodies associated with lupus erythematosus. Science. 1981; **211**(4480):400-402

[27] Ben-Chetrit E, Gandy BJ, Tan EM, Sullivan KF. Isolation and characterization of a cDNA clone encoding the 60-kD component of the human SS-A/Ro ribonucleoprotein autoantigen. The Journal of Clinical Investigation. 1989;**83**(4):1284-1292

[28] Yamagata H, Akizuki M, Tojo T, Homma M. Anti-Ro/SSA and -La/SSB antibodies in patients with connective tissue diseases. Scandinavian Journal of Rheumatology. Supplement. 1986;**61**:98-101

[29] Dugar M, Cox S, Limaye V, et al. Diagnostic utility of anti-Ro52 detection in systemic autoimmunity. Postgraduate Medical Journal. 2010;**86**:79-82

[30] Lee LA, Farris AD. Photosensitivity diseases: Cutaneous lupus erythematosus. The Journal of Investigative Dermatology. Symposium Proceedings. 1999;**4**(1):73-78

[31] Yoshimi R, Ueda A, Ozato K, Ischigatsubo Y. Clinical and pathological roles of Ro/SSA autoantibody system. Clinical & Developmental Immunology. 2012;**2012**:606195. DOI: 10.1155/2012/606195 Epub 2012 Dec 6

[32] Yoshimi R, Ishigatsubo Y, Ozato K. Autoantigen TRIM21/Ro52 as a possible target for treatment of systemic lupus erythematosus. International Journal of Rheumatology. 2012;**2012**:718237. DOI: 10.1155/2012/718237 Epub 2012 Jun 4

[33] Montano-Loza AJ, Shums Z, Norman GL, Czaja AJ. Prognostic implications of antibodies to Ro/SSA and soluble liver antigen in type 1 autoimmune hepatitis. Liver International. 2012;**32**(1):85-92

[34] Rao L, Liu G, Li C, et al. Specificity of anti-SSB as a diagnostic marker for the classification of systemic lupus erythematosus. Experimental and Therapeutic Medicine. 2013; **5**:1710-1714

[35] Arbuckle MR, McClain MT, Rubertone MV, et al. Development of autoantibodies before the clinical onset of systemic lupus erythematosus. The New England Journal of Medicine. 2003;**349**:1526-1533

[36] Ingegnoli F, Castelli R, Gualtierotti R. Rheumatoid factors: Clinical applications. Disease Markers. 2013;**35**(6):727-734

[37] Simard JF, Holmqvist M. Rheumatoid factor positivity in the general population. British Medical Journal. 2012;**345**:e5841

[38] Tasliyurt T, Kisacik B, Kaya SU, et al. The frequency of antibodies against cyclic citrullinated peptides and rheumatoid factor in healthy population: A field study of rheumatoid arthritis from northern Turkey. Rheumatology International. 2013;**33**(4):939-942

[39] Witte T, Hartung K, Sachse C, et al. Rheumatoid factors in systemic lupus erythematosus: Association with clinical and laboratory parameters. SLE study group. Rheumatology International. 2000;**19**(3):107-111

[40] Bournia VK, Diamanti KD, Vlachoyiannopoulos PG, Moutsopoulos HM. Anticentromere antibody positive Sjögren's Syndrome: A retrospective descriptive analysis. Arthritis Research & Therapy. 2010;**12**(2):R47. DOI: 10.1186/ar2958. Epub 2010

[41] Salliot C, Gottenberg JE, Bengoufa D, Desmoulins F, Miceli-Richard C. Mariette Anticentromere antibodies identify patients with Sjögren's syndrome and autoimmune overlap syndrome. The Journal of Rheumatology. 2007;**34**(11):2253-2258

[42] Ho KT, Reveille JD. The clinical relevance of autoantibodies in scleroderma. Arthritis Research & Therapy. 2003;**5**(2):80-93

[43] Bencimon C, Salles G, Moreira A, et al. Prevalence of anticentromere F protein autoantibodies in 347 patients with non-Hodgkin lymphoma. Annals of the New York Academy of Sciences. 2005;**1050**:319-326

[44] Briasoulis E et al. CENP-B specific anti-centromere autoantibodies heralding small-cell lung cancer. A case study and review of the literature. Lung Cancer. 2008;**60**:302-306

[45] Atalay C, Dogan L, Atalay G. Anti-CENP-B antibodies are associated with prolonged survival in breast cancer. Future Oncology. 2010;**6**(3):471-477

[46] Bournia VK, Vlachoyiannopoulos PG. Subgroups of Sjögren syndrome patients according to serological profiles. Journal of Autoimmunity. 2012;**39**(1-2):15-26

[47] Payet J, Goulvestre C, Bialé L, et al. Anticyclic citrullinated peptide antibodies in rheumatoid and nonrheumatoid rheumatic disorders: Experience with 1162 patients. The Journal of Rheumatology. 2014;**41**(12):2395-2402. DOI: 10.3899/jrheum.131375 Epub 2014 Oct 1

[48] He J, Ding Y, Feng M, Guo J, Sun X, Zhao J, Yu D, Li Z. Characteristics of Sjögren's syndrome in rheumatoid arthritis. Rheumatology (Oxford, England). 2013;**52**(6):1084-1089. DOI: 10.1093/rheumatology/kes374 Epub 2013 Feb 4

[49] Lundberg K, Bengtsson C, Kharlamova N, et al. Genetic and environmental determinants for disease risk in subsets of rheumatoid arthritis defined by the anti-citrullinated protein/peptide antibody fine specifity profile. Annals of the Rheumatic Diseases. 2014; **73**:652-658

[50] Nezos A, Cinoku I, Mavgrani CP, Mautsopoulos HM. Antibodies against citrullinated alpha enolase peptides in primary Sjogren's syndrome. Clinical Immunology. 2017; **183**:300-303. DOI: 10.1016/j.clim.2017.09.012 Epub 2017 Sep 14

[51] Shen L, Suresh L, Lindemann M, et al. Novel autoantibodies in Sjogren's syndrome. Clinical Immunology. 2012;**145**:251-255

[52] De Langhe E, Bossuyt X, Shen L, Malyavantham K, Ambrus JL, Suresh L. Evaluation of autoantibodies in patients with primary and secondary Sjogren's syndrome. Open Rheumatology Journal. 2017;**11**:10-15

[53] Vishwanath S, Everett S, Shen L, Malyavantham K, Suresh L, Ambrus JL. Xerophthalmia of Sjogren's syndrome diagnosed with anti-salivary gland protein 1 antibodies. Case Reports in Ophthalmology. 2014;**5**(2):186-189

[54] Park K, Park S, Jackson MV. The inhibitory effects of muscarinic autoantibodies in the sera of primary Sjögren's syndrome patients on the gastrointestinal motility. Molecular Immunology. 2013;**56**:583-587

[55] Kovacs L, Marczinovitis I, Gyorgy A, Toth GK, Dorgai L, Pol J, Molnar J, Pokorny G. Clinical associations of autoantibodies to human muscarinic acetylocholine receptor 3 in primary Sjogren's syndrome. Rheumatology. 2005;**44**:1021-1025

[56] Iizuka M, Wakamatsu E, Tsuboi H, et al. Pathogenic role of immune response to M3 muscarinic acetylcholine receptor in Sjögren's syndrome-like sialoadenitis. Journal of Autoimmunity. 2010;**35**(4):383-389

[57] Dawson L, Tobin A, Smith P, Gordon T. Antimuscarinic antibodies in Sjögren's syndrome. Where are we, and where are we going? Arthritis & Rheumatism. 2005;**52**(10):2984-2995

[58] Verkman AS, Mitr AK. Structure and function of aquaporin water channels. American Journal of Physiology. Renal Physiology. 2000;**278**:F13-F28

[59] Delporte C, Steifeld S. Distribution and roles of aquaporins in salivary glands. Biochimica et Biophysica Acta. 2006;**1758**:1061-1070

[60] Tsubota K, Hirai S, King LS, Agre P, Ishida N. Defective cellular trafficking of lacrimal gland aquaporin-5 in Sjögren's syndrome. Lancet. 2001;**357**(9257):688-689

[61] Tzartos JS, Stergiou C, Daoussis D, Zisimopoulou P, Andonopoulos AP, Zolota V, Tzartos SJ. Antibodies to aquaporins are frequent in patients with primary Sjögren's syndrome. Rheumatology (Oxford). 2017;**56**(12):2114-2122. DOI: 10.1093/rheumatology/kex328

[62] Chauvin S, Sobel A. Neuronal stathmins: A family of phosphoproteins cooperating for neuronal development, plasticity and regeneration. Progress in Neurobiology. 2015; **126**:1-18. DOI: 10.1016/j.pneurobio.2014.09.002 Epub 2014 Oct 16

[63] Duda S, Witte T, Stangel M, Adams J, Schmidt RE, Baerlecken NT. Autoantibodies binding to stathmin-4: New marker for polyneuropathy in primary Sjögren's syndrome. Immunologic Research. 2017;**65**(6):1099-1102

[64] Qin Q, Wang H, Wang HZ, Huang YL, Li H, Zhang WW, Zhang JR, He LL, Xia R, Zhao DB, Deng AM. Diagnostic accuracy of anti-alpha-fodrin antibodies for primary Sjögren's syndrome. Modern Rheumatology. 2014;**24**(5):793-797. DOI: 10.3109/14397595.2013.865823. Epub 2013 Dec 29

[65] Ruffatti A, Ostuni P, Grypiotis P, Botsios C, Tonello M, Grava C, Favaro M, Todesco S. Sensitivity and specificity for primary Sjögren's syndrome of IgA and IgG anti-alpha-fodrin antibodies detected by ELISA. The Journal of Rheumatology. 2004;**31**(3):504-507

[66] Sordet C, Gottenberg JE, Goetz J, et al. Anti-α-fodrin autoantibodies are not useful diagnostic markers of primary Sjögren's syndrome. Annals of the Rheumatic Diseases. 2005;**64**:1244-1245

[67] Hernández-Molina G, Nuñez-Alvarez C, Avila-Casado C, et al. Usefulness of IgA anti-α-fodrin antibodies in combination with rheumatoid factor and/or antinuclear. Antibodies as substitute immunological criterion in Sjögren syndrome with negative anti-SSA/SSB antibodies. The Journal of Rheumatology. 2016;**43**(10):1852-1857

[68] Cui L, Elzakra N, Shuaimei X, Xiao GG, Yang Y, Hu S. Investigation of three potential autoantibodies in Sjogren's syndrome and associated MALT lymphoma. Oncotarget. 2017;**8**(18):30039-30049

Chapter 8

Autoantibodies in Silicosis Patients: Silica-Induced Dysregulation of Autoimmunity

Suni Lee, Hiroaki Hayashi, Naoko Kumaga-Takei,
Hidenori Mastzaki, Kei Yoshitome, Nagisa Sada,
Masayasu Kusaka, Kozo Uragami,
Yasumitsu Nishimura and Takemi Otsuki

Additional information is available at the end of the chapter

http://dx.doi.org/10.5772/intechopen.72999

Abstract

Silica particles cause silicosis (SIL) and represent one of the most typical environmental and occupational substances that induce autoimmune disorders among the exposed population. Anti-nuclear antibody (ANA), anti-Sjögren's-syndrome-related antigen A (SS-A), anti-centromere protein B (CENP)-B, and anti-scleroderma (Scl)-70 autoantibodies were examined in SIL and compared with those in healthy volunteers (HV) and patients with systemic sclerosis (SSc). Individuals with SIL were prone to autoimmune diseases and some autoantibodies seemed to be important as an estimation of this condition. Anti-Fas autoantibody found in SIL was functionally capable of inducing apoptosis in Fas-expressing cells, and this may cause a decrease of regulatory T cells (Tregs) expressing Fas in SIL. Moreover, responder T cells (Tresps) in SIL seemed to be activated chronically and protected from Fas-mediated apoptosis. Thus, an imbalance of Tresps (dominant) and Tregs (less) occurred in SIL. All of these causes of SIL are ready to further develop autoimmune diseases.

Keywords: silicosis, anti-CENP-B autoantibody, anti-Fas autoantibody, apoptosis, regulatory T cell, responder T cell

1. Introduction

Many environmental and occupational substances such as vinyl chloride, epoxy resins, solvents, pesticides, paraffin/silicone and silica particles cause dysregulation of autoimmunity [1, 2]. Silica-exposed patients suffer from silicosis (SIL), a condition that is well known to complicate with various autoimmune diseases [3, 4]. Of course, silica exposure produces typical pneumoconiosis [5, 6], which is defined as lung inflammation and fibrosis with scarring in the form of nodules in the middle to upper lungs. Although various clinical types such as acute, progressive and chronic SIL are distinguished depending on the exposed dosage of silica particles and duration, patients clinically exhibit dyspnea, fatigue, cough, chest pain and other pulmonary symptoms. There are several typical pulmonary complications such as pulmonary tuberculosis, tuberculous pleurisy, pneumothorax, bronchiectasis and lung cancer [7, 8].

In addition to these lung complications, it is well known that the condition of SIL patients is often complicated with autoimmune diseases. The classical disease is known as Caplan's syndrome, complicated with rheumatoid arthritis (RA) [9]. The initial description reported by Caplan involved 51 cases among coal miners. Thereafter, many epidemiological reports revealed high odds ratios for the occurrence of RA in SIL [10, 11]. Furthermore, other autoimmune diseases such as systemic sclerosis (SSc) [12, 13], systemic lupus erythematosus (SLE) [14, 15] and anti-neutrophil cytoplasmic antibody (ANCA) positive vasculitis/nephritis [16, 17] have been reported in case reports and epidemiological investigations.

We have been studying the direct effects of silica particles on human lymphocytes, especially responder T (Tresp) and regulatory T (Treg) cells [18–20], as well as investigating autoantibodies found in SIL [21–28]. In this chapter, clinical evaluation, epitope search and functional assays of several autoantibodies found in SIL are described and mechanistic analyses of T cells exposed to silica particles are conducted.

2. Anti-CENP-B and Scl-70 autoantibodies

The clinical evaluation of anti-centromere protein B (CENP-B) and scleroderma (Scl)-70 autoantibodies in SIL patients was performed and reported [29].

Figure 1 shows the titers of anti-nuclear antibody (ANA), anti-Sjögren's-syndrome-related antigen A (SS-A) antibody (Ab), anti-CENP-B and anti-Scl-70 (also known as anti-topoisomerase I) Abs in healthy volunteers (HV), SIL and SSc. All subjects were Japanese. 19 HV [median age = 46.0 years old (y.o.); mean ± standard deviation (SD) = 44.8 ± 8.6 y.o.; male:female (M:F) = 8:11], 20 SIL [median age = 73.5 y.o.; mean ± SD = 74.9 ± 5.4; male:female (M:F) = 19:1] and 25 SSc [median age = 65.0 y.o.; mean ± SD = 62.3 ± 12.1; male:female (M:F) = 3:22] were included in the study. All SIL were brickyard workers in Bizen City, Okayama prefecture, Japan, and were diagnosed according to the ILO 2000 guideline for pneumoconiosis. They were clinically followed in Kusaka Hospital or Hinase Uragami Iin according to Japanese law regarding the medical care of pneumoconiosis patients. The amount of free silica inhaled by these patients was estimated as high as 40 to 60% as determined from the work environment. These individuals did not show any symptoms of autoimmune diseases such as sclerotic skin, Raynaud's phenomenon, facial erythema or arthralgia. The SSc patients were diagnosed and monitored by the Department of Dermatology, Kawasaki Medical School Hospital, Kurashiki, Japan [29].

As shown in **Figure 1A**, investigation of the titers of ANA in HV, SIL and SSc revealed that a few SIL cases showed a higher titer of ANA, but there was no statistical significance. Not surprisingly, most of the SSc cases showed significantly higher ANA (compared to HV and SIL). Interestingly, titers of anti-Sjögren's-syndrome-related antigen A (SS-A) in SIL and SSc were higher than those of HV (**Figure 1B**). SS-A may be detected not only in Sjögren's syndrome, but also in other autoimmune diseases such as SSc and SLE. However, it may be interesting to note that SIL without any symptoms related to autoimmune diseases exhibited a higher titer for anti-SS-A Ab. Although clinical evaluation of anti-SS-A Ab in SIL has not been investigated, it is worth mentioning that SIL showed a pre-clinical status for autoimmune diseases as indicated by various epidemiological studies [9–17].

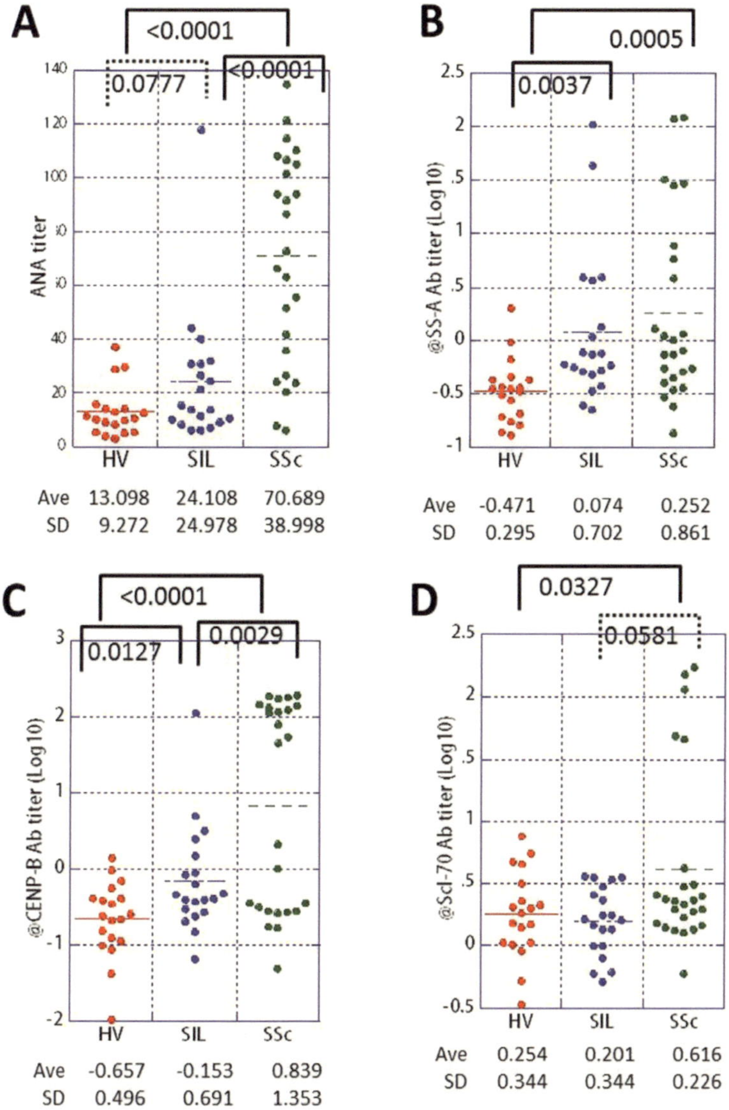

Figure 1. Comparison of titers for anti-nuclear antibody (ANA), anti-SS-A antibody (Ab), anti-CENP-B Ab and anti-Scl-70 Ab among healthy volunteers (HV), silicosis cases (SIL) and patients with systemic sclerosis (SSc). Except for ANA, titers are shown as logarithmic values. Statistical significance was examined using the student T-test and $p < 0.05$ was defined as significant. All titers were measured using a multiplex ELISA kit for ANA.

The evaluation of SSc showed that anti-CENP-B and anti-Scl-70 Abs were typical autoantibodies. Anti-CENP-B Ab is usually thought to be found in SSc cases with a type of localized skin lesion. On the other hand, SSc cases positive for anti-Scl-70 Ab are regarded as a generalized type with diffuse and extensive skin lesions [30–32]. Our results shown in **Figure 1C** (anti-CENP-B Ab) and **1D** (anti-Scl-70 Ab), for both Abs, demonstrated that there were clear breaks between positive and negative (close to levels of HV) cases in SSc. Regarding SIL, anti-CENP-B Ab was significantly higher than that in HV with the highest case whose titer was just as high as the positive case in SSc [29]. However, there was no case that showed higher anti-Scl-70 Ab in this series of SIL cases [29].

Thus, the clinical evaluation of anti-CENPN Ab in SIL was performed [29]. There was no correlation with other immunological or respiratory parameters in SIL such as titer of ANA, immunoglobulin (Ig) G, Ig A, Ig M, age, radiological classification of SIL (PR: profusion ratio), exposure years, percentage vital capacity (VC), forced expiratory volume 1.0 (SEC) (FEV1.0 (%)) or forced expiratory flow at 25% of vital capacity divided by body height (V25/H) except positive for anti-Scl-70 Ab titers, although anti-Scl-70 titers were similar to the those of HV. Factor analysis was performed using these immunological and respiratory clinical parameters [29]. As a result, anti-CENP-B Ab was found to contribute to the second and fourth factors. Factor 2 (17.7% contribution ratio) comprised the titer indices of anti-CENP-B and Scl-70 Abs, Ig G and age, all with positive values. This factor is understood as an immunological factor with aged patients showing a tendency for higher antibodies and Ig G. The fourth factor with a 13.2% contribution ratio was formed by the titer index of anti-CENP-B Ab with a negative value, the anti-Scl-70 autoantibody with a positive value, in addition to the Ig A level with a positive value. As found in the analyses of individual correlations, the titer index of anti-Scl-70 Ab and Ig A showed a positive correlation. This fourth factor indicated that even though the titer index of anti-Scl-70 autoantibody was located in the range of HV, among these titers, there is a correlation with Ig A and this tendency was the opposite of that observed for the titer index of anti-CENP-B auto-Ab. Thus, even with lower levels of titers, higher SIL cases with anti-CENP-B or anti-Scl-70 Ab differed as both Abs were divided in subtypes of SSc. Taken together, both Abs, especially anti-CENP-B (as well as anti-SS-A Ab), may indicate a pre-clinical status for forthcoming manifestations of autoimmune disease in SIL [29].

3. Autoantibodies against apoptosis-related molecules

Our previous reports indicated that autoantibodies against molecules related to apoptosis, Fas and caspase-8, were found in SIL [26–28]. These molecules may be expressed when cells in the body progressed to apoptosis in physiological as well as pathological situations.

Regarding anti-caspase-8 auto-Ab, although HV and cases comprised a different series from the aforementioned volunteers and cases, anti-caspase-8 auto-Ab was detected in 70% of HV, 62% of SIL, 90% of SSc and 60% of SLE cases, using four fragments of caspase-8 protein [26]. As a result, the positivity was not unique to autoimmune diseases and SIL. It was easily detected even in sera of HV. The report that revealed these positivities for anti-caspase-8 auto-Ab examined the epitope mapping. The epitopes were widely spread from the death effector domain to caspase regions and there was no specific epitope expressed in specific disease types such as SSc, SLE, SIL or HV [26].

http://dx.doi.org/10.5772/intechopen.72999

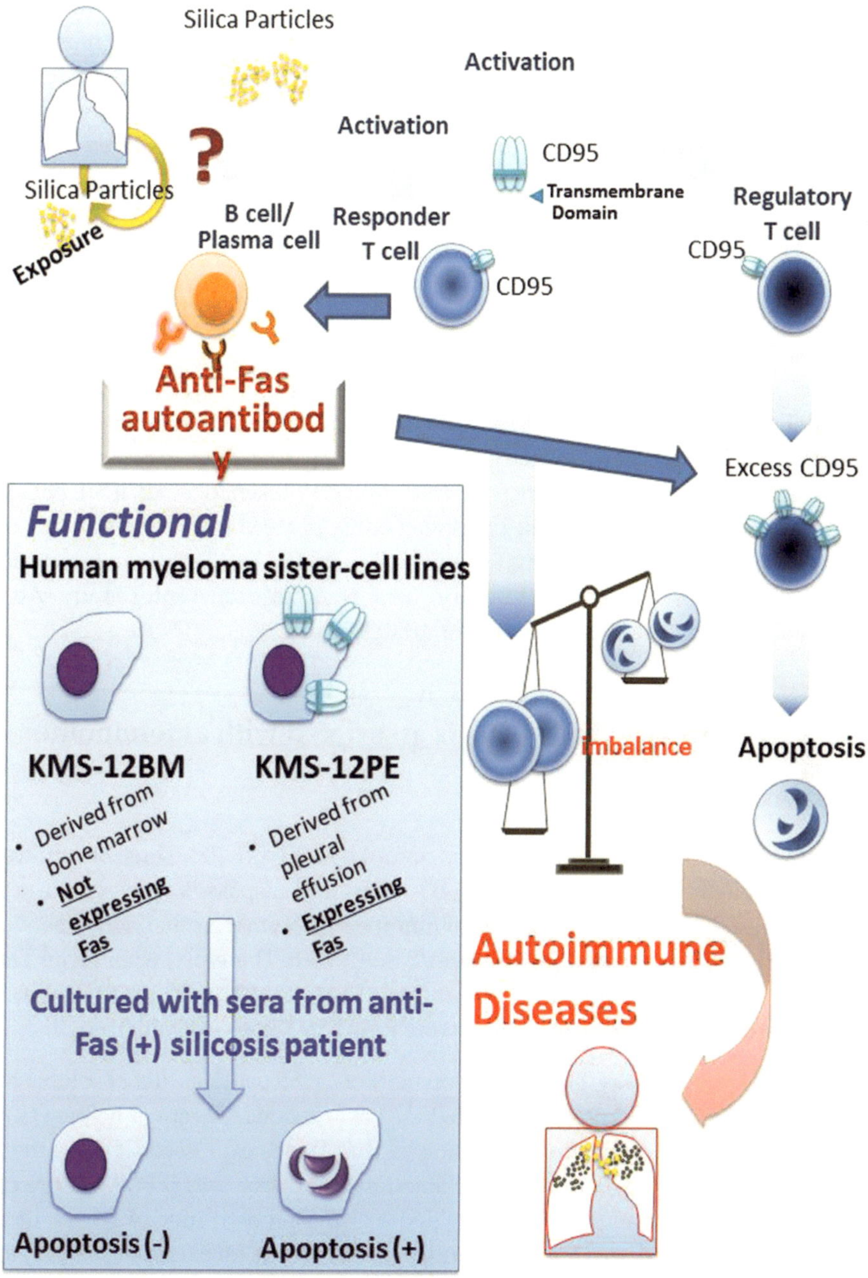

Figure 2. Anti-Fas auto-Ab was found in ca. 25% of SIL. The function of anti-Fas auto-Ab was examined using sister human myeloma cell lines, KMS-12PE and KMS-12BM. Only Fas-expressing KMS-12PE proceeded onto apoptosis when cultured with sera from SIL which revealed the highest titer for anti-Fas auto-Ab. Since anti-Fas auto-Ab seems to be functional, regulatory T cells (Tregs) in SIL with this auto-Ab may fall into apoptosis, given the higher expression of Fas in Tregs from SIL compared to responder T cells (Tresps) from SIL or Tregs from HV. As a result, an imbalance of Tresps (dominant) and Tregs (less) will occur.

The anti-Fas auto-Ab was also found in SIL cases [28]. This was detected as 23.1% in SIL, 53.3% in SLE and 46.7% in SSc, but not detected in HV. For the anti-Fas auto-Ab, epitope mapping was also performed and there was no special site, with epitopes being widely spread from the cysteine-rich domain (CRD) in extracellular sites to the death domain in intracellular sites. However, in contrast to anti-caspase-8 auto-Ab (caspase-8 is an intracellular molecule), anti-Fas-auto-Ab can bind to the Fas molecule which is present on the cell surface and, if this auto-Ab is functional, cells presenting Fas/death receptor may be induced toward apoptosis. Thus, we examined whether anti-Fas auto-Ab is functional, whereby it can cause cell death and growth inhibition in Fas-expressing cells [28]. For this purpose, two myeloma cell lines established in our laboratory, called KMS-12PE and KMS-12BM, were employed which were sister cell lines derived from the same Japanese myeloma patients [33]. KMS-12PE was derived from an earlier stage of patients and from pleural effusion, while KMS-12BM was derived from the terminal stage and from bone marrow. Interestingly, Fas expression was higher in KMS-12PE, but very scant in KMS-12BM [28, 33]. Thus, we incubated both cell lines with sera from SIL which showed the highest titer for anti-Fas auto-Ab. As a result, KMS-12PE progressed to apoptosis, but 12BM did not [28]. From these analyses, anti-Fas auto-Ab functions to induce apoptosis against Fas-expressing cells. From our previous study [34], it was found that Tregs in SIL expressed higher levels of Fas molecules compared to Tregs derived from HV. Taken together, if SIL patients possessed anti-Fas auto-Ab in their serum, Tregs may easily proceed to apoptosis and be reduced [34]. The imbalance of Tregs and Tresps (dominant Tresps and less Tregs) is a typical situation that induces the occurrence of autoimmune disorders. Thus, functional anti-Fas auto-Ab is a key molecule involved in dysregulation of autoimmunity (**Figure 2**).

4. Other autoantibodies and silicosis associated with autoimmune diseases

Some reports have identified anti-desmoglein auto-Ab in SIL [21, 22]. Thus, SIL showed various auto-Abs against ANA, Scl-70, CENP-B, SS-A, Fas and caspase-8. How are these various auto-Abs manifested in SIL without any autoimmune symptoms? As mentioned above, Tregs may be reduced in SIL, especially SIL with anti-Fas auto-Ab. Therefore, what about Tresps? If the imbalance defined by dominant Tresps and less Tregs is important for the onset of autoimmune diseases, what kinds of alterations were found in Tresps derived from SIL?

We found that there were many T cell activation markers in SIL, such as higher soluble interleukin (IL)-2 receptor [34], higher program death (PD)-1 expression in Tresps (T helper (Th) 4 cells) as well as Tregs [35], and an *in vitro* assay showed that Tresps expressed CD69 as the earliest activation marker of T cells when peripheral blood mononuclear cells (PBMCs) were cultured with silica particles [36]. In addition to this evidence of chronic activation of Tresps, there were many inhibitors of Fas-mediated apoptosis present in SIL serum, for example, soluble Fas (sFas) [37] and Fas-alternatively spliced variants (lacking the transmembrane domain, but maintaining the Fas-ligand binding domain) [38]. Additionally, PBMCs from SIL showed higher decoy receptor 3 (DcR3; which acts similar to sFas binding with trail-apoptosis induced at the extracellular area) expression compared to PBMCs from HV [39] (**Figure 3**). Taken together, Tresps in SIL are stimulated and survive longer by inhibition of Fas-mediated apoptosis. These Tresps can encounter various self-antigens and force B cells to produce auto-Abs [18–20].

http://dx.doi.org/10.5772/intechopen.72999

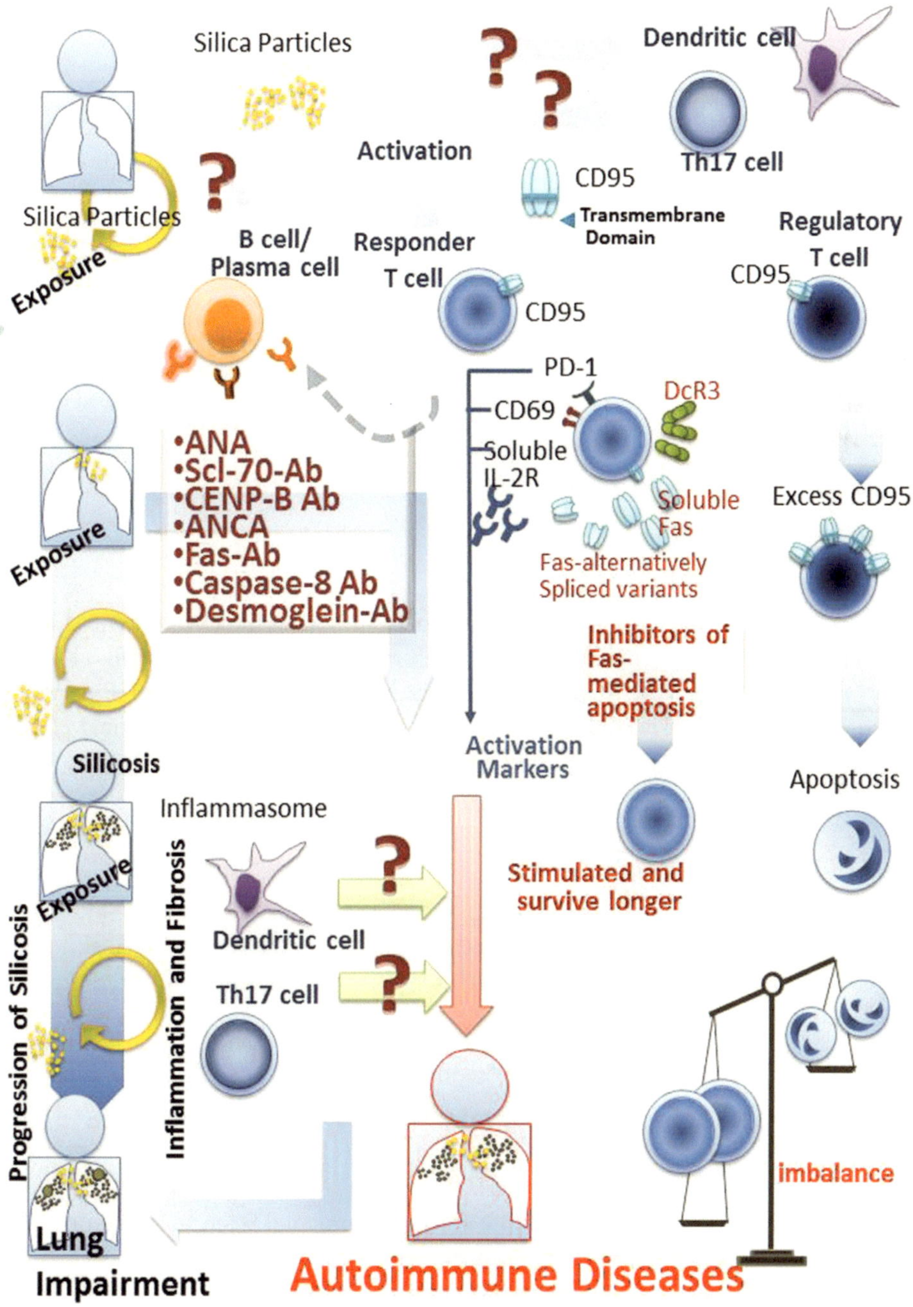

Figure 3. In addition to various auto-Abs found in SIL, and earlier apoptosis of Tregs in SIL, Tresps in SIL revealed a chronically activated status with CD69 and PD-1 expression as well as higher serum soluble IL-2 receptor. Additionally, Tresps in SIL inhibited Fas-mediated apoptosis by excess soluble Fas and similar molecules such as DcR3. Thus, Tresps in SIL survive longer and encounter various autoantigens. Moreover, the imbalance between Tresps and Tregs may be enhanced.

5. Conclusion

SIL is prone to autoimmune diseases. SIL patients were positive for various auto-Abs such as ANA, SS-A, CENP-B and Fas. Some auto-Abs possess certain clinical values that reflect pre-autoimmune status. These auto-Abs are produced from B cells/plasma cells that receive some commands to generate these Abs from T cells. In T cells in SIL, an imbalance exists between Tresps and Tregs. Both are chronically activated by long-term silica exposure. Thereafter, Tresps survive longer and Tregs proceed to apoptosis. However, the cytokine status in SIL needs to be examined and compared with HV as well as some autoimmune diseases, SSC, SLE or ANCA-related vasculitis. Additionally, the role and alteration of Th17 cells require investigation from the viewpoint of autoimmune diseases, since these are considered to be important in modifying autoimmune status and dendritic cells which initially recognize silica particles.

Acknowledgements

The authors appreciate the assistance of former colleagues from the Department of Hygiene, Kawasaki Medical School, Kurashiki, Japan, Professor Ayako Ueki, Drs. Yasuhiko Kawakami, Fuminori Hyodoh, Akiko Takata-Tomokuni, Yoshie Miura, Shuko Murakami, Ping Wu, Ying Chen and Megumi Maeda. The authors are also grateful for technical support from Ms. Yumika Isozaki, Haruko Sakaguchi, Tamayo Hatayama, Shoko Yamamoto and Miho Ikeda.

Author details

Suni Lee[1], Hiroaki Hayashi[2], Naoko Kumaga-Takei[1], Hidenori Mastzaki[3], Kei Yoshitome[1], Nagisa Sada[1,4], Masayasu Kusaka[5], Kozo Uragami[6], Yasumitsu Nishimura[1] and Takemi Otsuki[1]*

*Address all correspondence to: takemi@med.kawasaki-m.ac.jp

1 Department of Hygiene, Kawasaki Medical School, Kurashiki, Okayama, Japan

2 Department of Dermatology, Kawasaki Medical School, Kurashiki, Okayama, Japan

3 Department of Life Science, Faculty of Life and Environmental Science, Prefectural University of Hiroshima, Shobara, Hiroshima, Japan

4 Department of Biophysical Chemistry, Graduate School of Medicine, Dentistry and Pharmaceutical Sciences, Okayama University, Okayama, Japan

5 Kusaka Hospital, Nishikatagami, Bizen, Okayama, Japan

6 Hinase Uragami Iin, Hinase, Hinase-Town, Bizen, Okayama, Japan

References

[1] Haustein UF, Anderegg U. Silica induced scleroderma – Clinical and experimental aspects. The Journal of Rheumatology. 1998;**25**:1917-1926

[2] Hess EV. Environmental chemicals and autoimmune disease: Cause and effect. Toxicology. 2002;**181-182**:65-70

[3] Pollard KM. Silica, silicosis, and autoimmunity. Frontiers in Immunology. 2016;**7**:97. DOI: 10.3389/fimmu.2016.00097

[4] Steenland K, Goldsmith DF. Silica exposure and autoimmune diseases. American Journal of Industrial Medicine. 1995;**28**:603-608

[5] Wagner GR. Asbestosis and silicosis. Lancet. 1997;**349**:1311-16315

[6] Castranova V, Vallyathan V. Silicosis and coal workers' pneumoconiosis. Environmental Health Perspectives. 2000;**108**(Suppl 4):675-684

[7] Balaan MR, Weber SL, Banks DE. Clinical aspects of coal workers' pneumoconiosis and silicosis. Occupational Medicine. 1993;**8**:19-34

[8] Hnizdo E, Vallyathan V. Chronic obstructive pulmonary disease due to occupational exposure to silica dust: A review of epidemiological and pathological evidence. Occupational and Environmental Medicine. 2003;**60**:237-243

[9] Caplan A. Certain unusual radiological appearances in the chest of coal-miners suffering from rheumatoid arthritis. Thorax. 1953;**8**:29-37

[10] Sluis-Cremer GK, Hessel PA, Hnizdo E, Churchill AR. Relationship between silicosis and rheumatoid arthritis. Thorax. 1986;**41**:596-601

[11] Klockars M, Koskela RS, Järvinen E, Kolari PJ, Rossi A. Silica exposure and rheumatoid arthritis: A follow up study of granite workers 1940-81. British Medical Journal (Clinical Research Ed.). 1987;**294**:997-1000

[12] Rodnan GP, Benedek TG, Medsger TA, Jr Cammarata RJ. The association of progressive systemic sclerosis (scleroderma) with coal miners' pneumoconiosis and other forms of silicosis. Annals of Internal Medicine. 1967;**66**:323-334

[13] Sluis-Cremer GK, Hessel PA, Nizdo EH, Churchill AR, Zeiss EA. Silica, silicosis, and progressive systemic sclerosis. British Journal of Industrial Medicine. 1985;**42**:838-843

[14] Costallat LT, De Capitani EM, Zambon L. Pulmonary silicosis and systemic lupus erythematosus in men: A report of two cases. Joint, Bone, Spine. 2002;**69**:68-71

[15] Yamazaki S, Yoshiike F, Hirai K, Kakegawa T, Ikeda M, Nagata A, Saito G, Nishimura H, Hosaka N, Ehara T. Silica-associated systemic lupus erythematosus in an elderly man. Internal Medicine. 2007;**46**:1867-1871

[16] Tervaert JW, Stegeman CA, Kallenberg CG. Silicon exposure and vasculitis. Current Opinion in Rheumatology. 1998;**10**:12-17

[17] Bartůnková J, Pelclová D, Fenclová Z, Sedivá A, Lebedová J, Tesar V, Hladíková M, Klusácková P. Exposure to silica and risk of ANCA-associated vasculitis. American Journal of Industrial Medicine. 2006;**49**:569-576

[18] Lee S, Hayashi H, Mastuzaki H, Kumagai-Takei N, Otsuki T. Silicosis and autoimmunity. Current Opinion in Allergy and Clinical Immunology. 2017;**17**:78-84. DOI: 10.1097/ACI.0000000000000350

[19] Lee S, Matsuzaki H, Kumagai-Takei N, Yoshitome K, Maeda M, Chen Y, Kusaka M, Urakami K, Hayashi H, Fujimoto W, Nishimura Y, Otsuki T. Silica exposure and altered regulation of autoimmunity. Environmental Health and Preventive Medicine. 2014;**19**:322-329. DOI: 10.1007/s12199-014-0403-9

[20] Maeda M, Nishimura Y, Kumagai N, Hayashi H, Hatayama T, Katoh M, Miyahara N, Yamamoto S, Hirastuka J, Otsuki T. Dysregulation of the immune system caused by silica and asbestos. Journal of Immunotoxicology. 2010;**7**:268-278. DOI: 10.3109/1547691X.2010.512579

[21] Ueki H, Kohda M, Hashimoto T, Komai A, Nobutoh T, Yamaguchi M, Ohmori K, Miyashita F, Yoda N. Bullous pemphigoid associated with silicosis. Dermatology. 2000;**201**:265-267

[22] Ueki H, Kohda M, Nobutoh T, Yamaguchi M, Omori K, Miyashita Y, Hashimoto T, Komai A, Tomokuni A, Ueki A. Antidesmoglein autoantibodies in silicosis patients with no bullous diseases. Dermatology. 2001;**202**:16-21

[23] Ueki A, Isozaki Y, Tomokuni A, Tanaka S, Otsuki T, Kishimoto T, Kusaka M, Aikoh T, Sakaguchi H, Hydoh F. Autoantibodies detectable in the sera of silicosis patients. The relationship between the anti-topoisomerase I antibody response and HLA-DQB1*0402 allele in Japanese silicosis patients. Science of the Total Environment. 2001;**270**:141-148

[24] Ueki A, Isozaki Y, Tomokuni A, Ueki H, Kusaka M, Tanaka S, Otsuki T, Sakaguchi H, Hyodoh F. Different distribution of HLA class II alleles in anti-topoisomerase I autoantibody responders between silicosis and systemic sclerosis patients, with a common distinct amino acid sequence in the HLA-DQB1 domain. Immunobiology. 2001;**204**:458-465

[25] Tomokuni A, Otsuki T, Sakaguchi H, Isozaki Y, Hyodoh F, Kusaka M, Ueki A. Detection of anti-topoisomerase I autoantibody in patients with silicosis. Environmental Health and Preventive Medicine. 2002;**7**:7-10. DOI: 10.1007/BF02898059

[26] Ueki A, Isozaki Y, Tomokuni A, Hatayama T, Ueki H, Kusaka M, Shiwa M, Arikuni H, Takeshita T, Morimoto K. Intramolecular epitope spreading among anti-caspase-8 autoantibodies in patients with silicosis, systemic sclerosis and systemic lupus erythematosus, as well as in healthy individuals. Clinical and Experimental Immunology. 2002;**129**:556-561

[27] Ueki A, Isozaki Y, Kusaka M. Anti-caspase-8 autoantibody response in silicosis patients is associated with HLA-DRB1, DQB1 and DPB1 alleles. Journal of Occupational Health. 2005;**47**:61-67

[28] Takata-Tomokuni A, Ueki A, Shiwa M, Isozaki Y, Hatayama T, Katsuyama H, Hyodoh F, Fujimoto W, Ueki H, Kusaka M, Arikuni H, Otsuki T. Detection, epitope-mapping and function of anti-Fas autoantibody in patients with silicosis. Immunology. 2005;**116**:21-29

[29] Lee S, Hayashi H, Kumagai-Takei N, Matsuzaki H, Yoshitome K, Nishimura Y, Uragami K, Kusaka M, Yamamoto S, Ikeda M, Hatayama T, Fujimoto W, Otsuki T. Clinical evaluation of CENP-B and Scl-70 autoantibodies in silicosis patients. Experimental and Therapeutic Medicine. 2017;**13**:2616-2622. DOI: 10.3892/etm.2017.4331

[30] Domsic RT. Scleroderma: The role of serum autoantibodies in defining specific clinical phenotypes and organ system involvement. Current Opinion in Rheumatology. 2014;**26**: 646-652. DOI: 10.1097/BOR.0000000000000113

[31] Pollard KM, Reimer G, Tan EM. Autoantibodies in scleroderma. Clinical and Experimental Rheumatology. 1989;**7**(Suppl 3):S57-S62

[32] Jabłońska S, Błaszczyk M, Jarzabek-Chorzelska M, Chorzelski T, Kołacińska-Strasz Z. Immunological markers of the subsets of systemic scleroderma and its overlap. Archivum Immunologiae et Therapiae Experimentalis (Warsz). 1991;**39**:381-390

[33] Ohtsuki T, Yawata Y, Wada H, Sugihara T, Mori M, Namba M. Two human myeloma cell lines, amylase-producing KMS-12-PE and amylase-non-producing KMS-12-BM, were established from a patient, having the same chromosome marker, t(11,14)(q13;q32). British Journal of Haematology. 1989;**73**:199-204

[34] Hayashi H, Miura Y, Maeda M, Murakami S, Kumagai N, Nishimura Y, Kusaka M, Urakami K, Fujimoto W, Otsuki T. Reductive alteration of the regulatory function of the CD4(+)CD25(+) T cell fraction in silicosis patients. International Journal of Immunopathology and Pharmacology. 2010;**23**:1099-1109

[35] Hayashi H, Maeda M, Murakami S, Kumagai N, Chen Y, Hatayama T, Katoh M, Miyahara N, Yamamoto S, Yoshida Y, Nishimura Y, Kusaka M, Fujimoto W, Otsuki T. Soluble interleukin-2 receptor as an indicator of immunological disturbance found in silicosis patients. International Journal of Immunopathology and Pharmacology. 2009;**22**:53-62

[36] Wu P, Hyodoh F, Hatayama T, Sakaguchi H, Hatada S, Miura Y, Takata-Tomokuni A, Katsuyama H, Otsuki T. Induction of CD69 antigen expression in peripheral blood mononuclear cells on exposure to silica, but not by asbestos/chrysotile-a. Immunology Letters. 2005;**98**:145-152

[37] Tomokuni A, Otsuki T, Isozaki Y, Kita S, Ueki H, Kusaka M, Kishimoto T, Ueki A. Serum levels of soluble Fas ligand in patients with silicosis. Clinical and Experimental Immunology. 1999;**118**:441-444

[38] Otsuki T, Sakaguchi H, Tomokuni A, Aikoh T, Matsuki T, Isozaki Y, Hyodoh F, Kawakami Y, Kusaka M, Kita S, Ueki A. Detection of alternatively spliced variant messages of Fas gene and mutational screening of Fas and Fas ligand coding regions in peripheral blood mononuclear cells derived from silicosis patients. Immunology Letters. 2000;**72**:137-143

[39] Otsuki T, Tomokuni A, Sakaguchi H, Aikoh T, Matsuki T, Isozaki Y, Hyodoh F, Ueki H, Kusaka M, Kita S, Ueki A. Over-expression of the decoy receptor 3 (DcR3) gene in peripheral blood mononuclear cells (PBMC) derived from silicosis patients. Clinical and Experimental Immunology. 2000;**119**:323-327

Chapter 9

Indicators of Preeclampsia in Correlation with Maternal Cytokines in Pregnancy

Ana Daneva Markova, Marija Hadzi-Lega,
Goran Dimitrov, Gligor Tofovski,
Jadranka Georgievska, Elena Dzikova and Ivo Kjaev

Additional information is available at the end of the chapter

http://dx.doi.org/10.5772/intechopen.76344

Abstract

Aim: the purpose of the actual study was to evaluate, in the third trimester of pregnancy, the relationship between the formation of anti-inflammatory IL-10 cytokine and several indicators of moderate and severe preeclampsia. Materials and methods: in the third trimester of gestation, examination of the biochemical markers of preeclampsia (PE) and maternal IL-10 levels was conducted in 100 women with pregnancies complicated by varying degrees of preeclampsia and in 100 normotensive patients, hospitalized at the University Clinic of Gynecology and Obstetrics, Skopje, Republic of Macedonia. Patients with preeclampsia were categorized into moderate and severe preeclampsia groups according to the degree of preeclampsia. Logistic regression of the different parameters for the occurrence of severe preeclampsia analysis was used to determine the predictive value. Results: the regression analysis detected systolic blood pressure of 160 mmHg or higher, diastolic blood pressure of 100 mmHg or higher, persistent proteinuria in pregnancy, serum LDH concentration of 450 U/L or higher, and reduced serum concentrations of IL-10 as significant predictors of severe preeclampsia. Conclusion: significantly, lower IL-10 concentrations in maternal serum in patients with severe preeclampsia in comparison with respective concentrations in patients with moderate preeclampsia can be considered as major pathognomonic laboratory sign of severe form of preeclampsia.

Keywords: cytokines, indicators, preeclampsia, biochemical markers, prediction

1. Introduction

Preeclampsia (PE), one of the current problems of obstetrics, is a pathological multifactorial syndrome that occurs in the second half of pregnancy and is manifested through a basic triad of symptoms: swelling, proteinuria, and hypertension and in severe cases, convulsions and coma [1, 2]. Preeclampsia remains one of the most sophisticated problems of modern obstetrics and gynecology. It generally determines the structure of maternal and perinatal morbidity and mortality. The role of immune mechanisms contributing to the development of a normal pregnancy is widely discussed. Their involvement in the pathogenesis of pregnancy complications such as preeclampsia was also noted [3]. The analysis of the scientific literature reveals the conclusion that many aspects of the pathogenesis of preeclampsia are related with systemic inflammatory response syndrome with the development of a destructive inflammatory process, immune disorders, and the imbalance of cytokine regulation of gestation processes [4–6].

The role of vascular endothelial damage with the development of generalized arteriolar spasm as one of the leading mechanisms in the pathogenesis of preeclampsia is supposed to be significant. However, the relationship between the development of endothelial dysfunction and disruption of cytokine regulation in different clinical forms of preeclampsia also requires further research and is currently represented in several scientific works [7].

Proteinuria has been proposed and studied as both an indicator of the severity of the disease and a predictor of the outcome in preeclampsia. Many clinicians still make major management decisions based on the degree of proteinuria in these patients.

Cytokines, such as IL-2, IL-8, and TNF-α, are pro-inflammatory, increased in the blood, in leukocytes during PE. Elevated concentrations of TNF-α have been observed in the blood of women with PE [8]. Further studies support the idea of the involvement of the maternal immune system in the development of preeclampsia which comes from the prim paternity theory [9]. This hypothesis holds that the risk of developing preeclampsia is highest in the first pregnancy [10], and a previous normal pregnancy is associated with a lowered incidence of preeclampsia [11] in the subsequent pregnancy.

In contrast to normal pregnancy, there are indications of increased inflammatory responses [12] and also of an immune deviation toward Th1 in the established preeclampsia pregnancy [13]. Roberts et al. [14] were one of the first to suggest that mediators released in preeclampsia are responsible for the endothelial damage seen in preeclampsia. Subsequent to the damage, the injured endothelium initiates a dysfunctional cascade of coagulation, vasoconstriction, and intravascular fluid redistribution that results in the clinical syndrome of preeclampsia [15].

Numerous studies show that the balance of cytokines has special importance in the regulation of pregnancy. However, the diagnostic and prognostic significance of breaches in the immune balance during preeclampsia has not yet been determined.

2. Aim

The purpose of the actual study was to evaluate the relationship between the formation of anti-inflammatory cytokines and several indicators of moderate and severe preeclampsia in the third trimester of pregnancy.

3. Materials and methods

We conducted a prospective study of 50 women with pregnancies complicated by varying degrees of preeclampsia in the third trimester of gestation with singleton pregnancies between 28 and 40 weeks' gestation (±1 week), parity (parity 1 1–4 and parity > 4), and maternal age (<20 years, 20–35, and >35 years) and in 50 normotensive patients without threatening signs of hypertension and preeclampsia, hospitalized at the University Clinic of Gynecology and Obstetrics, Skopje, Republic of Macedonia.

The severity of preeclampsia was determined according to the definition of the *WHO Handbook for Guideline Development*, Geneva, 2010. Our inclusion criteria were reproductive age, diagnosed moderate and severe preeclampsia based on the criteria for classification at the time of collection of maternal serum, and the patients' informed consent for inclusion in the survey.

Exclusion criteria were acute and chronic genital and extra genital diseases (essential hypertension, heart failure, diabetes, morbid obesity, immunodeficiency, systemic diseases, chronic infectious diseases, genetic pathology).

Patients with preeclampsia were categorized into moderate (m PE) group A and severe (S PE) preeclampsia group B according to the degree of preeclampsia.

Cytokine levels in the serum were measured by the "sandwich" method of solid-phase enzyme immunoassay using double antibody. As a standard for comparison of each reaction, recombinant cytokines were used, which are part of the test—whale.

Statistical data processing was done using the SPSS 13.0 software for Windows.

4. Results

Regarding patients' distribution by ethnicity, in **Table 1**, Albanians represented more than half of the women with preeclampsia as 44% of participants with symptoms of medium and 68% with symptoms of severe PE. Pregnant Albanians (68%) dominate in the group with normal tension.

The average body mass index (BMI) in the group of pregnant women with preeclampsia was 34.33 ± 4.5—that was not significantly higher than tile average body mass of the control group (32.88 ± 3.8) ($p = 0.09$). The difference between the average BMI of pregnant women with moderate and severe PE and normotensive patients was significant ($F = 3.8$, $p = 0.026$). Namely, pregnant women with severe PE had significant higher average BMI than normotensive pregnant women (35.57 ± 4.11 vs. 32.88 ± 3.8, $p = 0.025$).

Statistical analysis is showed, not significant differences in the levels of interleukin 10 in serum between pregnant women with preeclampsia and healthy pregnant women ($p = 0.5$), but the difference between moderate preeclampsia, severe preeclampsia, and control group was highly significant ($p < 0.01$) due to the lower levels of this interleukin in the severe preeclampsia group comparing moderate preeclampsia in relation to the control and due to the significant lower values when comparing control in relation to the moderate preeclampsia

Variable	Groups			
	All PE	**Moderate PE**	**Severe PE**	**Control (C)**
	N = 50	N = 25	N = 25	N = 50
Age (years)	32.06 ± 4.8	29.9 ± 4.7	34.2 ± 3.85	31.8 ± 4.8
mean ± SD				
All PE/C t = 0.27 p = 0.8				
mPE/sPE/C; F = 5.5; p = 0.005		**post hoc mPE/sPE p = 0.004**		
Gestational week, mean ± SD	34.99 ± 3.5	35.5 ± 3.4	34.4 ± 3.6	34.8 ± 3.6
All PE/C; t = 0.2; p = 0.8				
mPE/sPE/C F = 0.6 p = 0.5				
Ethnicity n %				
Macedonian	18 (36%)	10 (40%)	8 (32%)	15 (30%)
Albanian	28 (56%)	11 (44%)	17 (68%)	34 (68%)
Romani	4 (8%)	4 (16%)	0	1 (2%)
BMI mean ± SD, range	34.33 ± 4.5	33.1 ± 4.7	35.57 ± 4.1	32.88 ± 3.8
	24.2–44	24.2–41	27–44	27–43.9
All PE/C; t = 1.7; p = 0.09				

Table 1. Age, gestational week, BMI, and IL-10 serum concentration in women with moderate and severe preeclampsia, and women with normal blood pressure (control group).

group. Average concentrations of IL-10 in serum were 23.2 ± 40.7 pg/ml in the total group of preeclampsia patients, 45.5 ± 48.4 pg/ml in the group with moderate preeclampsia, and 0.8 ± 0.4 pg/ml in the group with severe preeclampsia. In patients with normal tension, the average serum concentration of interleukin 10 was 4.2 ± 6.7 pg/ml.

Study data demonstrated that in pregnant women with pregnancy complicated by preeclampsia, the serum concentration of anti-inflammatory interleukin 10 is confirmed as a significant predictor of the occurrence of severe preeclampsia (**Table 2**). Increased serum concentrations of interleukin 10 (in pg/ml) reduced the likelihood of the development of severe preeclampsia by 89.6% (95% CI 0.016–0.678).

Figures 1–3 show that the results of bivariate analysis are of the relationships between serum maternal concentration of IL-10 and serum enzyme LDH, creatinine, platelets, proteinuria, and uric acid.

The obtained values of Pearson's coefficients indicate negative correlations of interleukin 10 with LOH and proteinuria, whereas the correlations of IL-10 with creatinine platelets and uric acid were positive. However significant correlations were confined between interleukin 10 and platelets as well as between IL-10 and proteinuria. The correlation with the platelet count was positive which means that significantly higher concentration of interleukin 10 was confirmed in patients with higher number of platelets in the blood and vice versa. The correlation between interleukin

Variable	B	S.E.	Wald	Sig.	Exp(B)	95.0% CI for Exp(B)	
Age	0.2	0.086	5.350	0.021	1.221	1.031	1.446
Nulliparity (present)	1.816	1.114	2.657	0.103	6.145	0.692	54.534
Systolic blood pressure (≥160 mmHg)	3.711	1.053	12.412	0.000	40.900	5.189	322.371
Diastolic blood pressure (≥100 mmHg)	2.414	0.843	8.192	0.004	11.176	2.140	58.360
Proteinuria (present)	3.081	1.307	5.56	0.018	21.785	1.682	282.123
LDH ≥ 450 (U/L)	2.066	0.915	5.102	0.024	7.896	1.314	47.433
Albumin (serum) (g/L)	−0.239	0.125	3.66	0.056	0.787	0.616	1.006
Creatinine (serum) (umol/L)	−0.067	0.035	3.696	0.055	0.935	0.873	1.001
Platelets (≤150)	−0.006	0.013	0.236	0.627	0.994	0.97	1.019
IL-10 (pg/ml)	−2.324	1.051	4.888	0.027	0.098	0.012	0.768

Dependent variable: severe preeclampsia.

Table 2. Multivariate logistic regression analysis for the factors predictors of severe preeclampsia.

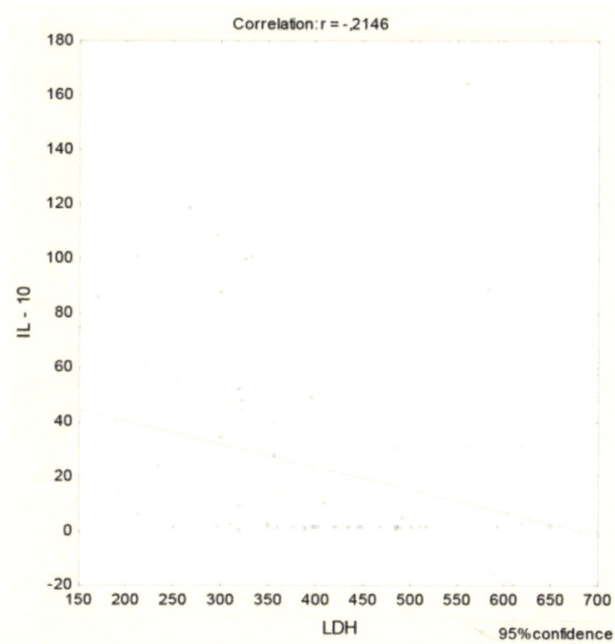

Figure 1. Correlation IL-10/LDH: r = −0.215 and p = 0.134.

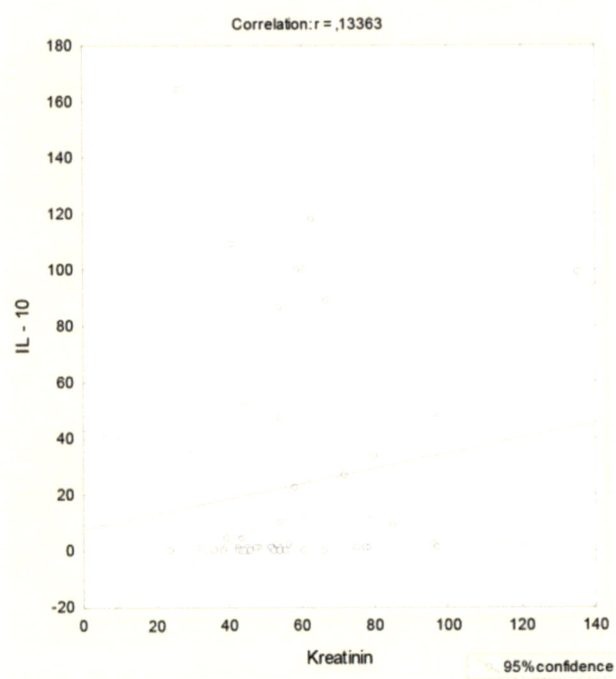

Figure 2. Correlation IL-10/creatinine: r = 0.134 and p = 0.355.

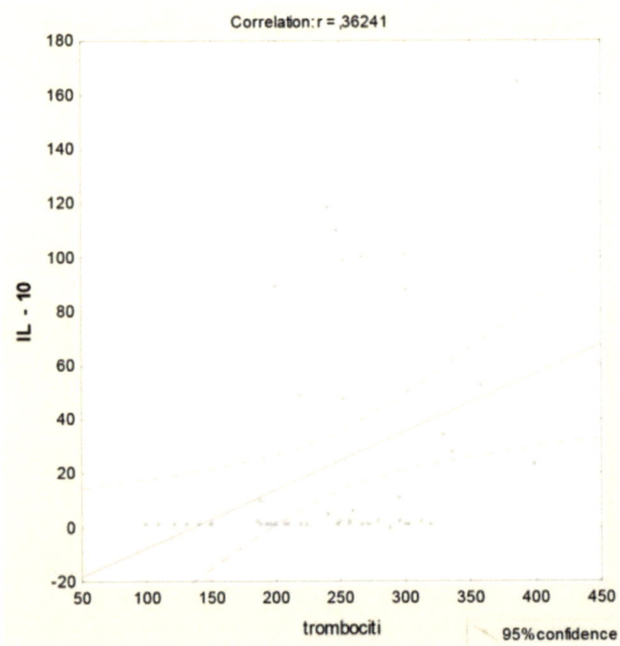

Figure 3. Correlation IL-10/platelets.

10 and proteinuria was negative showing that the serum concentration of interleukin 10 was significantly lower in patients with higher amount of proteins in the urine and vice versa.

5. Discussion

This study demonstrates differences in IL-10 levels in women with preeclampsia compared to the levels in women with a normal pregnancy outcome.

We found that in pregnant women with preeclampsia the increased serum concentrations of IL-10 predicted lower likelihood for the development of severe preeclampsia.

Longitudinal studies in mice demonstrate a sequential change in the cytokine profile in serum including interleukin 10 in peripheral blood and release from spleen elements as pregnancy advances.

In the second half of pregnancy, IL-10 inhibition in mice is related with fetal growth retardation [16]. Progesterone has been shown to increase Th2-type responses in T cells [17]. This study demonstrated that there is a significant alteration in the serum concentration of IL-10 in severe preeclampsia compared with normal pregnancy and in moderate preeclampsia groups of patients.

The regression analysis applied in this study showed diastolic blood pressure of 100 mmHg or higher, systolic blood pressure of 160 mmHg or higher, persistent proteinuria in pregnancy, the serum LDH concentration of 450 U/L or higher, and reduced serum concentrations of IL-10 in maternal serum as significant predictors of severe preeclampsia. While other variables predicted the development of severe preeclampsia, IL-10 decreased such likelihood. IL-10 was also found to be negatively correlated with proteinuria and positively correlated with blood platelets. Significantly higher concentration of IL-10 was confirmed in patients with higher number of platelets in the blood. The serum concentration of IL-10 was significantly lower in patients with higher amount of proteins in the urine.

This study demonstrated platelet count and proteinuria as significant predictors of serum IL-10 concentration—urine proteins predicting lower serum IL-10 while platelets count predicting higher serum concentration of interleukin 10.

Other studies suggest a proportional link between the level of proteinuria and adverse clinical outcomes. In recent study 13,000 pregnant women found significant proteinuria, defined as 21 or more on dipstick analysis, and it was associated with an increase in prematurity rates, intrauterine fetal growth restriction, and increased neonatal morbidity and mortality when associated with hypertension [18]. Other studies suggest that it is the presence of proteinuria rather than the severity, which is associated with poorer outcomes in these complications for mother and stillbirth. There is evidence that even the finding of trace proteinuria in pregnant women with hypertension is associated with an increase in adverse outcomes.

Taking into consideration changes of anti-inflammatory cytokine concentrations in severe preeclampsia, the moderate phase can be analyzed as a critical stage in complicated pregnancy.

6. Conclusion

Cytokines play critical, essential roles in signaling between cells of the immune system, with a prolific range of regulatory activities including the stimulation, recruitment, activation, destroying, and suppression of immune and nonimmune cells.

Analyzing cytokines at the end of pregnancy, last trimester complicated with preeclampsia, is useful. The moderate phase can be considered a critical stage in preeclampsia that comes to the most functional strain homeostatic system.

Abbreviation

BMI	body mass index
PE	preeclampsia
TNF-α	tumor necrosis factor-α

Author details

Ana Daneva Markova[1,2*], Marija Hadzi-Lega[1], Goran Dimitrov[1], Gligor Tofovski[1], Jadranka Georgievska[1], Elena Dzikova[1] and Ivo Kjaev[1]

*Address all correspondence to: anadaneva@yahoo.com

1 Medical Faculty, University Clinic of Obstetrics and Gynecology, Ss. Cyril and Methodius University, Skopje, Macedonia

2 Department of Obstetrics and Gynecology, State University Hospital of Skopje, Skopje, Macedonia

References

[1] Vikhlyaeva M. Preclinical manifestations of systemic disorders. Clinical outcomes and long term effects of preeclampsia. Obstetrics and Gynecology. 2009;**1**:3-6

[2] Tsatsaris V, Fournier T, Winer N. Pathophysiology of preeclampsia. European Joumal of Obstetrics & Gynecology and Reproductive Biology. 2008;**1**:16-23

[3] Sukhin GT, Vanko LV. Immune factors in the etiology and pathogenesis of pregnancy complications. Obstetrics and Gynecology. 2012;**1**:128-136

[4] Lewis DF, Canzoneri BJ, Wang Y. Maternal circulating TNF-alpha levels are highly correlated with IL-10 levels but not IL-6 and IL-8 levels in women with pre-eclampsia. American Journal of Repirodnctive lmmunology. 2009;**5**:269-274

[5] Kalkunte S, Nevers T, Norris WE, Sharma S. Vascular IL-10: A protective role in preeclampsia. Journal of Reproductive Immunology; **88**:165-169

[6] Tosun M, Celik H, Avci B, Yavuz E, Alper T, Malatyalioglu E. Maternal and umbilical serum levels of interleukin-6. Interleukin −8. and tumor necrosis factor-alpha in normal pregnancies and in pregnancie complicated by preeclampsia. Journal of Maternal - Fetal and Neonatal Medicine. 2010;**23**:880-886

[7] Molvarec A, Szarka A, Walentin S, Beko G, Karádi I, Prohászka Z, Rigó J Jr. Serum leptin levels in relation to circulating cytokines. Chemokines. Adhesion molecules and angiogenic factors in normal pregnancy and preeclampsia. Reproductive Biology and Endocrinology. 2011;**9**:124-133

[8] Bosio PM, PJ MK, Conroy R, O'Herlihy C. Maternal central hemodynamics in hypertensive disorders of pregnancy. Obstet Gynecollogy. 1999;**94**:978-984

[9] Lim KH, Friedman SA, Ecker J, Kao L, Kilpatrick SJ. The clinical utility of serum uric acid measurements in hypertensive diseases of pregnancy. The American Journal of Obstetrics and Gynecology. 1998;**178**:1067-1071

[10] Makarov IO, Shemanaeva TV, Hasanov SR, Popova OP. Preeclampsia as a manifestation of immune endotheliosis. The Questions of Gynecology. Obstetrics and Perinatology. 2009;**6**:17-22

[11] Sidorova IS, Gurin OI, Milovanov AP. The pathogenesis of preeclampsia as a manifestation of immune-endothelial pathology (acute immune endothe- liosis). Obstetrics and Gynecology. 2008;**6**:13-17

[12] Hashii K, Flljiwara S, Yoshioka N, Kataoka S, Yamada T, Hirano T. Peripheral blood mononuclear cells stimulate progesterone production. By luteal cells derived from pregnant and non pregnant women: Possible involement of interleukin −4 and interleukin-10 in corpus luteum function.and dlifferentiation. Human Reproduction. 1998;**13**:2738

[13] Chaouat G, Meliani AA, Martal R, et al. IL-10 prevents naturally occurring fetal loss in the CBA 3 DBA/2 mating combination and local defect in IL-10 production in this abortion -prone combination is corrected by in vivo injection of IFN-γ. The Journal of Immunology. 1995;**154**:4261-4268

[14] Delassus S, Coutinho C, Saucier S, Darehe Kourilsky P. Differential cytoxine expression maternal blood and placenta during muringestation. The Journal of Immunology. 1994;**152**:2411

[15] Athanassakis I, Iconomidou B. Cytokine production in the serum and spleen of mice from day 6 to 14 of gestation: Cytokine/placenta/spleen/serum. Developmental Immunology. 1996;**4**:247

[16] Piccinni MP, Giudizi G, Biagotti R, Beloni L, Giannarini L. Progesterone favors the development of human T helper cells producing Th2 type cytokines and promotes both IL-4 production and membrane CD30 expression in established Th1 cell clones. The Journal of Immunology. 1995;**155**:128

[17] Rijhsinghani AG, Thompson K, Tygrette Bhatia SK. Inhibition of interleukin - 10 during pregnancy results in neonatal growth retardation. American Journal of Reproductive lmmunology. 1997;**37**:232

[18] Cote AM, Firoz T, Mattman A. The 24-hour urine collection: Gold standard or historical practice. The American Journal of Obstetrics and Gynecology. 2008;**1999**:625

Section 4

Autoantibodies Based Biomarker and their Assay

Chapter 10

Autoantibody-Based Diagnostic Biomarkers: Technological Approaches to Discovery and Validation

Farhanah Aziz, Muneera Smith and
Jonathan M Blackburn

Additional information is available at the end of the chapter

http://dx.doi.org/10.5772/intechopen.75200

Abstract

Autoantibodies produced against self-antigens, or 'autoantigens', result from a loss of self-tolerance triggered by genetic and/or environmental factors which induce the immune system to attack the host's own cells, resulting in a condition referred to as autoimmunity. In classic autoimmune diseases, it is well established that the pathology relates directly to the autoantibodies. However, it is increasingly recognised that autoantibodies are also found in many other disease areas, including cancers, cardiovascular and neurodegenerative diseases, as well infectious diseases such as malaria, albeit in such diseases it is unclear whether the autoantibodies play a direct role in the pathology or whether they are merely symptomatic of disease. Irrespective of whether they are causative or symptomatic of specific diseases though, there is increasing interest globally in exploring the clinical potential of circulating autoantibodies as diagnostic biomarkers. This chapter provides an overview of the diagnostic utility of autoantibody biomarkers in a range of disease areas and discusses their potential utility in disease staging, treatment monitoring and in prediction of immune-related adverse events. It also provides an overview of traditional and contemporary technological approaches to autoantibody biomarker discovery and validation, focusing on protein microarrays that are ideally suited to this important area of research.

Keywords: autoantibody biomarkers, protein microarrays, pre-symptomatic diagnosis, immune-related adverse events

1. Introduction

Autoantibodies are natural antibodies produced against self-antigens, or 'autoantigens', and can induce the immune system to attack host tissues, leading to a condition generically referred to as autoimmunity. Classic autoimmune syndromes include systemic lupus erythematosus, rheumatoid arthritis, rheumatic heart disease, Graves' disease, autoimmune hepatitis, multiple sclerosis, diabetes, and Sjogren's syndrome. In such autoimmune diseases, it is well established that the pathology relates directly to the autoantibodies. However, it is increasingly recognised that autoantibodies are also found in many other diseases, including cancers, cardiovascular diseases, neurodegenerative diseases, as well infectious diseases such as malaria, albeit in such diseases it is not yet clear whether the autoantibodies play a direct role in the pathology or whether they are merely symptomatic of disease. Irrespective of whether the autoantibodies are causative or symptomatic of specific diseases though, there is increasing interest globally in exploring the clinical potential of circulating autoantibodies as diagnostic biomarkers and considerable research effort is now being directed to the discovery, quantitation and validation of novel autoantibody-based diagnostic biomarkers in many different disease areas.

Numerous techniques have been utilised over the last few decades to detect the presence of autoantibodies in patient samples, not least since autoantibodies are increasingly thought to represent excellent potential biomarkers for early disease detection. Techniques that have historically been employed for biomarker identification include western blotting, immunohistochemistry and enzyme-linked immunosorbent assays (ELISA), but these are being superseded now by newer technologies that offer higher multiplicity as well as greater sensitivity and specificity. Amongst these newer technologies, protein microarrays are becoming established now as a powerful means to detect protein expression levels and to investigate protein-ligand interactions, as well as to probe protein function [1], since they enable efficient and sensitive, high throughput protein analysis, with large numbers of technically-replicated measurements being made in parallel using miniaturised assay formats and minimal sample volumes. These properties of protein microarrays make them ideally suited to component-resolve and quantify autoantibody profiles in biological samples.

2. Autoantibodies: a brief overview

2.1. Autoantibody classes

Antibodies are secreted heterodimeric proteins comprising light and heavy chains which are produced in mammals through recombination of V(D)J segments in developing B-lymphocytes. At any one time, there are thought to be of the order of 10^7–10^8 different antibody sequences present in human serum. In response to the presence of foreign antigens or pathogens, somatic hypermutation processes drive the affinity maturation of specific antibody sequences, resulting in the production of high affinity, antigen-specific antibodies. Affinity-matured antibodies, or immunoglobulins (Igs), are produced by plasma cells and secreted into the blood stream where they scavenge their cognate antigen for destruction. Antibodies thus play a crucial adaptive role in mammalian defence mechanisms against harmful components that can cause disease. There are five classes of antibodies: IgG, IgM, IgE, IgD and IgA, which differ in their structures and immune functions. IgG is the major antibody class found in blood, has the longest serum half-life of all immunoglobulin isotypes [2] and contributes directly to a neutralising immune response to extracellular pathogens and toxins. IgA is also involved in direct neutralisation of toxins, virus and bacteria; however, it concentrates particularly in mucosal surfaces. IgM, a pentameric immunoglobulin, is the largest of the antibody classes and is associated with a primary immune response; IgMs are therefore frequently used to diagnose acute exposure to an immunogen or pathogen [2]. IgD and IgE are found in trace amounts in the blood with short half-lives. IgD remains membrane-bound and is involved in regulation of cell activation while IgE is associated with hypersensitivity and allergic reactions [2]. Classical autoantibodies are typically IgMs and include: anti-nuclear antibodies (ANA), which bind to the nuclear membrane, nucleoplasm, nucleoli and nuclear organelles of cells [3]; rheumatoid factor (RF), which binds with relatively low affinity to the Fc region of IgGs and which is found in the serum of rheumatoid arthritis (RA) patients [4]; Anti-double-stranded DNA (dsDNA) antibodies, anti-Sm antibodies, antiphospholipid antibodies, anti-Ro, anti-ribonucleoprotein and anti-La Antibodies which are all frequently found in systemic lupus erythematosus (SLE) patients [4]; and Anti-Sjogren's syndrome A (SSA) and -B (SSB) antibodies, which are found in many patients with Sjogren's syndrome [4].

2.2. Causes of autoantibody production

In a normal immune response to a foreign antigen, professional antigen presenting cells - including dendritic cells, B-cells and macrophages – engulf and proteolyse the antigen and then present antigen-derived peptides on their cell surface in the form of major histocompatibility complexes; recognition of complexed peptides by a specific receptor on a T-cell then triggers the release of cytokines and chemokines, resulting in activation of that T-cell. Interaction between antigen-specific T- and B-cells subsequently leads to antigen-specific B-cell proliferation [1, 2]. A portion of those B-cells serve as memory cells, whilst the remainder act as effector cells that differentiate into antibody-producing plasma cells responsible for the production and release of antigen-specific antibodies [5].

Peripheral tolerance mechanisms usually ensure that self-reactive T- and B-cells (i.e. displaying T- or B-cell receptors for self-antigens) are suppressed. However, in certain circumstances, peripheral tolerance can be broken, resulting in proliferation of autoantigen-specific T- and B-cells. Simplistically, peripheral tolerance can be broken for a number of reasons, for example if the self-antigen is significantly over-expressed in a tissue or if neoantigens are somehow presented to the host immune system. Such neoantigens can include mutated peptide epitopes, aberrantly spliced or aberrantly post-translationally-modified epitopes, or new discontinuous epitopes resulting from misfolding of the antigen. Tolerance defects can also stem from the downregulation of regulatory T-cells (Tregs) [6], whilst chronic inflammatory responses are thought to facilitate the release and exposure of intracellular antigens to the immune system, resulting in autoantibody production in cancer patients [7], as well as increased vasculature permeability, allowing immune cell accumulation at the tumour site [8]. One consequence of loss of peripheral tolerance can be the production of self-antigen-specific autoantibodies.

As mentioned above, autoantigens may result from aberrant post-translationally modifications, including proteolysis, hydrolysis, phosphorylation and oxidation [9]. One such example occurs in RA, where patients produce autoantibodies against citrulline-modified proteins, themselves produced by the enzymatic action of peptidylarginine deiminases (PADs) - calcium-dependent enzymes that catalyse the post-translational hydrolysis of peptidylarginine to peptidylcitrulline. During inflammation, oxidative stress or apoptosis, PAD converts specific arginine residues on selected proteins into citrulline (a process often referred to as 'citrullination'), thereby producing neoepitopes that are recognised as non-self, dramatically altering immunogenicity and autoantibody production in RA patients [10].

Autoantibodies are also produced in response to the uncontrolled released of autoantigens during cell death processes. Maintenance of tissue homeostasis ordinarily takes place via clearance of apoptotic and altered cells through phagocytosis- or complement-dependent mechanisms, inhibition of inflammation, removal of misfolded proteins, and regulation of autoantibody-producing B cells [11]. However, when clearance mechanisms becomes compromised, dead cells accumulate and progress to secondary necrosis, releasing autoantigens as well as pro-inflammatory markers and thereby disrupting immune homeostasis [12] (**Figure 1**).

Autoantibody production thus has a multifactorial aetiology in which environmental and inherited factors interplay in determining the autoantibody profiles of an individual. Environmental factors associated with autoantibody production include drugs, toxins, chemicals from personal care products, and infections. Exposure to such agents can result in modification or mutation of chromosomal DNA sequences, potentially giving rise to altered gene- and protein expression (which can drive altered post-translational modifications), as well as to the expression of aberrantly-spliced or mutated form of proteins, all of which can result in the generation of neoantigens in the exposed tissue and hence to the production of specific autoantibodies. Furthermore, genetic predisposition or family history of autoimmune disorders also contributes to one-third of the risk of having increased autoantibody levels and various genome-wide association studies have shown that the production of autoantibodies in SLE [13], RA [14] and Multiple Sclerosis [15] is controlled by multiple loci.

Although the self-reactivity of autoantibodies can be harmful to host tissues, recent studies suggest that low-grade self-reactivity also occurs in healthy individuals, implying that certain autoantibodies may play a role in maintaining immune homeostasis [16] and in protecting against pathogenic processes, by activating innate and acquired immunity to maintain or restore health status [16]. Natural autoantibodies are predominantly of the IgM class, which makes sense since IgM is the first antibody to appear when the immune system is triggered in response to external antigenic exposure. By contrast, circulating naive IgMs arise without known immune exposure or vaccination [11] but have also been reported to recognise certain autoantigens in healthy adults as well as in newborn babies [17, 18].

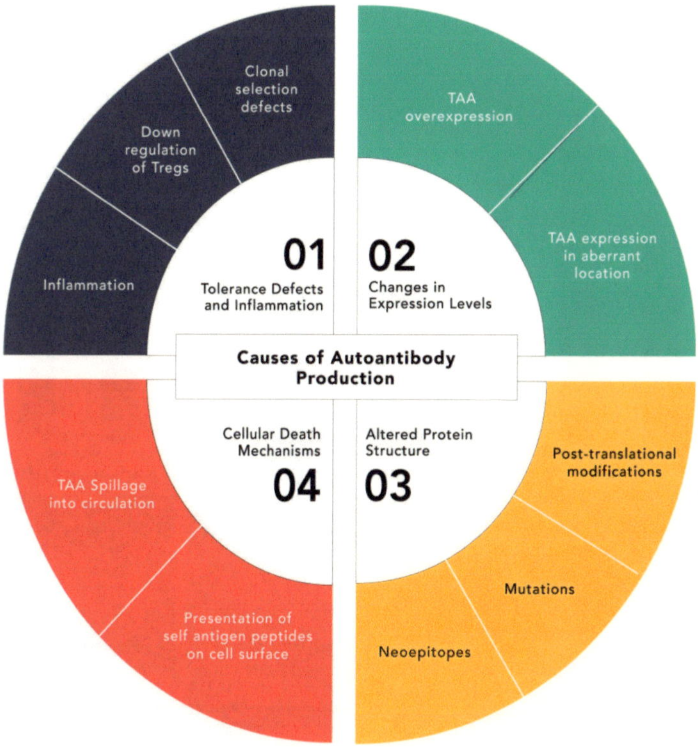

Figure 1. Key factors that increase antigenic pressure and cause the production of autoantibody in several diseases.

2.3. Gender bias in autoimmune diseases

The term 'autoimmune disease' refers to a group of over 80 distinct disorders, the symptoms and severity of which vary between individuals [19].

There are marked differences in diseases that predominantly affect males or females, as shown in **Figure 2**. Generally, females are more susceptible to autoimmune diseases whereas males show increased susceptibility to non-reproductive cancers. As females tend to have more responsive and robust immune system compared to their male counterparts, it is therefore not surprising that females respond more aggressively to autoantigens and are more susceptible to autoimmune diseases [20]. Other factors that contribute to the sex bias of autoimmune diseases include X-chromosomal abnormalities, X-chromosomal inactivation, and fetal micro-chimerism [20].

2.4. Functional role of autoantibodies in disease

The outcome of aberrant activation of the immune system and inflammatory process is dependent on multiple factors, including the type of affected tissue or organ and the degree of tissue injury sustained [21]. For example, in type 1 diabetes mellitus, the immune system reacts to insulin-producing cells in the pancreas. In other examples, tissues of the small intestines are

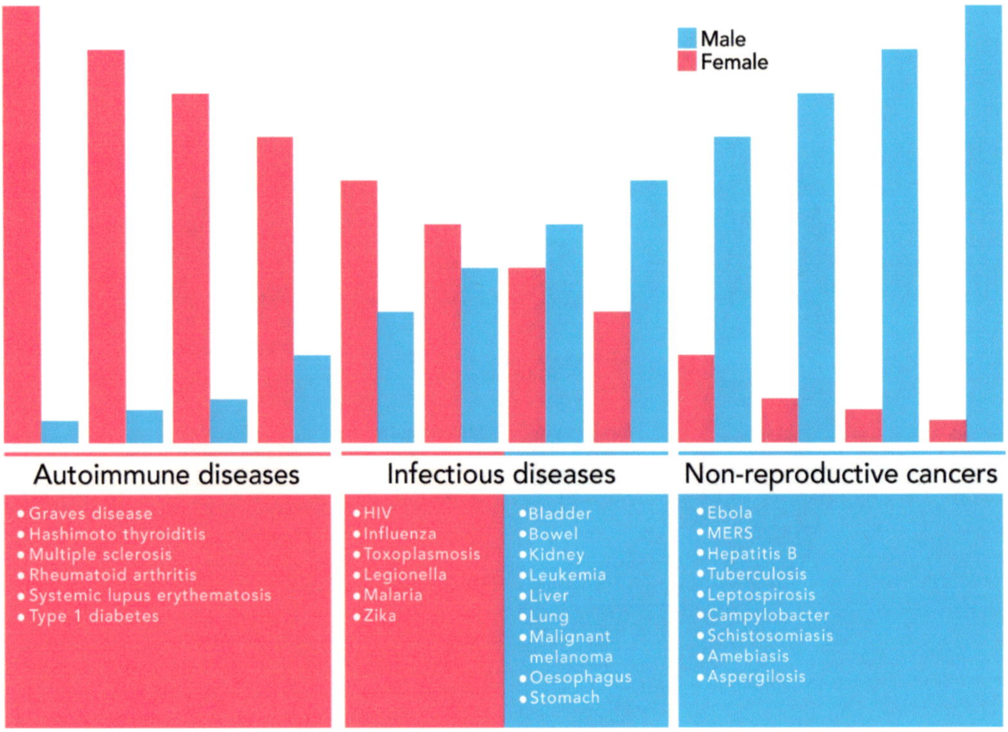

Figure 2. Gender-dependent susceptibility to autoimmune diseases, infectious diseases, inflammatory diseases and cancers.

affected in inflammatory bowel disease, while myelin - a fatty substance that protects nerve fibres in the brain and spinal cord - is destroyed in Multiple Sclerosis. In RA, connective tissues are affected and in SLE, auto-reactivity usually occurs in skin, heart and lung tissues. Sjogren's syndrome occurs when autoantibodies target secretory glands that produce tears and saliva, causing extreme dryness and other complications [22].

In other diseases, however, the functional role of autoantibodies is less clear. For example, in neurodegenerative diseases such as Parkinson's and Alzheimer's Diseases, increased cellular toxicity is caused by the accumulation and aggregation of misfolded proteins, which might also result in the generation of protective autoantibodies in some patients. For example, in Parkinson's Disease (PD), the protein alpha-synuclein misfolds and aggregates to form Lewy bodies; these bodies form in the brain tissues of PD patients and infiltrate the neurons, disrupting signalling process in the brain. A recent study reported that a defined set of epitopes derived from alpha-synuclein drive cytotoxic T-cell responses in people with PD [23], whilst another recent study reported a decline in anti-alpha-synuclein autoantibodies in PD patients compared to controls, suggesting that in some patients anti-alpha-synuclein autoantibodies might play a protective role [24].

Similarly, in Alzheimer's Disease (AD), the microtubule-associated protein Tau accumulates and aggregates in neurons causing neuronal degeneration. Tau also accumulates and aggregates in Progressive Supranuclear Palsy (PSP), a rare disease often misdiagnosed as Parkinson's disease. In AD, Tau causes misfolding of beta-amyloid, leading to amyloid-β (Aβ) plaque formation and downstream pathology, but in PSP, Tau itself mis-folds and agglomerates. These protein agglomerations subsequently leave the cell, spread throughout the brain and disrupt the communication between neurons [25]. Interestingly, a recent study identified an anti-Aβ plaque autoantibody in certain aged but cognitively firm individuals that was absent in AD patients; this autoantibody was cloned and has been shown to selectively target aggregated Aβ in a mouse model of AD, where it bound parenchymal Aβ and reduced soluble and insoluble Aβ in a dose-dependent manner; in Phase 2 clinical trials, this autoantibody, Aducanumab, reduced brain Aβ in patients with mild AD, again in a dose-dependent manner [26], strongly suggesting that anti- Aβ autoantibodies play a protective role in healthy individuals.

In cancers, chronic inflammation is a well-recognised hallmark and it is known that both cancer and autoimmune diseases can occur in the same individual, albeit in cancer, the immune response is often suppressed and unable to eliminate altered self-cells, while in autoimmune diseases it is hyper-activated against specific autoantigens. The act of manipulating the immune system in different ways, however, suggests a possible link between these two conditions [21] and it seems likely that inflammatory processes drives both autoimmunity and malignancy. However, it remains unclear whether it is the underlying autoimmunity that leads to malignancy ("inflammation-induced cancer") or whether the immune responses directed against tumour antigens lead to autoimmune diseases ("tumour-induced autoimmunity").

3. Diagnostic utility of autoantibody biomarkers

3.1. Early detection of disease

Autoantibody production is a key indicator of many diseases and has emerged as an important tool in predicting onset of a number of diseases. Autoantibodies are in principle detectable many years before manifestation of disease or symptoms and have been observed in an ever-widening range of disease areas, which makes novel autoantibodies attractive plausible biomarkers for early diagnosis of a broader spectrum of diseases now. Known autoantibody biomarkers have been reported to predate symptoms in Sjogren's syndrome, rheumatoid arthritis, Alzheimer's disease and cancers, as discussed below:

Sjogren's syndrome is an autoimmune disease that affects parts of the body which produce secretions such as tears and saliva. The symptoms overlap with other autoimmune conditions and can range from mild to severe, causing nausea, fatigue, joint pain as well as excessive dryness of the eyes and mouth. Autoantibodies attack cells in mucous membranes and moisture-secreting glands of the eyes and mouth, causing dryness, irritation and pain. A study published in 2015 concluded that autoantibodies are present up to 18–20 years before the diagnosis of primary Sjogren's syndrome [27]. A total of five autoantibodies were analysed, namely antinuclear antibodies, rheumatoid factor and autoantibodies against Ro 60/SSA, Ro

52/SSA, and La/SSB, with 81% of the patients who became seropositive after diagnosis having autoantibodies in pre-diagnostic serum samples. More importantly, these autoantibodies were present in the earliest available serum sample of 95% of the patients who expressed autoantibodies before diagnosis and before the onset of first symptoms [27].

RA is a chronic autoimmune disease characterised by inflammation of synovial joints, leading to joint erosion and deterioration. Rheumatoid factor and anti-cyclic citrullinated peptide (anti-CCP) are detected in the blood of 80% and 60–70% of RA-affected individuals, respectively. Anti-CCP autoantibodies were detected in some patient sera samples 12–14 years prior to the development of RA and 34–40% of the RA patients were anti-CCP positive prior to disease onset [28].

The presence of autoantibodies has also been implicated in AD. Aβ-autoantibodies were reported to show promise as an effective blood biomarker for AD and a positive association between Aβ-autoantibody titres and cognitive status have been reported [29]. Glial autoantibody markers to glutamate were detected in the plasma of AD patients and, interestingly, the level of that autoantibody in patients with moderate and severe dementia was 2-fold higher than that in patients with mild dementia [30]. In addition, autoantibodies to ATP synthase were reported to be found frequently in the sera of AD patients but not in age-matched healthy subjects or in patients with Parkinson's disease or atherosclerosis, suggesting anti-ATP synthase autoantibodies could be a specific biomarker for AD [29].

In addition to autoimmune diseases, multiple studies have described autoantibody production prior to cancer diagnosis, including in lung cancer [31], prostate cancer [32] and ovarian cancer [33]. Autoantibody production in cancer is thought to be a product of immunosurveillance - a process in which the body's own systems recognise and eliminate abnormal cells during early tumorigenesis [34] - suggesting that detection of disease-associated autoantibodies may be feasible in the asymptomatic stages of cancer and may predate the clinical signs of tumour progression by months or years, thus enabling their use in early diagnosis [35].

By way of example, in healthy mammalian cells, cAMP-dependent protein kinase A (PKA) is an intracellular enzyme, while in most cancers it is secreted into the circulatory system as ECPKA. The level of ECPKA was found to be elevated in various stages of a wide range of cancers including bladder, breast, cervical, colon, esophageal, gastric, liver, lung, ovarian, prostate, pancreatic, renal, small bowel, rectal, adenocystic carcinomas, melanoma, sarcoma, thymoma, liposarcoma, and leiomyosarcoma compared with healthy controls [35]. Extracellular protein kinase A (ECPKA) autoantibody is thus a potential serologic autoantibody for early-stage cancers diagnosis since it presents at high levels before surgical removal of solid tumours and diminishes after tumour removal [36]. An ELISA-based test for anti-ECPKA IgG was developed and the sensitivity and specificity of this biomarker for detecting 20 different cancers were reported to be 90 and 87% respectively, with the anti-ECPKA autoantibody being detected in 90% of the patient samples but in only 13% of the control samples [35].

Autoantibody-based screening for a variety of other cancers has also been carried out in laboratory environments. For example, Xie et al. developed a test platform by combining the detection of six autoantibodies directed against prostate cancer with PSA levels, increasing the accuracy of detection from 65% using PSA alone to 81% with both methods [37]. A similar outcome was achieved in breast cancer diagnosis using a panel of six autoantigens to detect ductal carcinoma *in situ* and lung cancer with specificity of 85 and 92%, respectively [38]. It is thus evident that having an increased level of specific circulating autoantibodies may reflect the overall state of the immune response of an individual, whilst the presence of such autoantibodies in otherwise healthy individuals might be an indicator of future autoimmune or other disorders.

3.2. Disease staging and treatment monitoring

An accurate pathology diagnosis is of central importance in precision medicine, since it should guide choice of the most effective treatment and management regimens. Reliable biomarkers for monitoring and prediction of disease course, stage and progression will be therefore invaluable, particularly in therapeutic decision-making to treat disease at an early stage. Current research has not only established the presence of autoantibodies in several diseases but has also shown that they have the potential to be used as biomarkers capable of diagnosis and staging various degrees of pathology. One such example is Type 1 insulin-dependent diabetes - a chronic autoimmune disease that impairs the insulin-producing beta cells in the pancreas, preventing the body from producing enough insulin to regulate blood glucose levels. This disease can be characterised into well-defined stages, and the rate of progression to symptomatic disease can be predicted with appreciable accuracy [39]. Stage 1 is defined by the presence of two or more islet autoantibodies and progressing at a variable rate to a second stage of glucose intolerance or dysglycaemia, before becoming clinically symptomatic (stage 3).

In another example, Cai et al. reported that anti-p53 antibodies develop several years before the clinical diagnosis of certain cancers and suggested that monitoring the change of serum p53 antibodies before and after treatment of patients diagnosed with oesophageal carcinoma with radiotherapy would be useful for evaluating the prognosis and response to the treatment. This study showed that the positive rate of p53-antibodies in patients with oesophageal carcinoma was related to histological grade, stage of the disease and lymph node metastasis but not to age, gender, or site of tumour formation. The study also reported a significant difference in the level of serum p53 antibodies before and after radiotherapy treatment, with the positive rate of p53 antibodies in patients who responded to radiotherapy being much lower than the patients who did not respond to radiotherapy [40]. A separate study by Shimada et al. showed that seropositive oesophageal squamous cell carcinoma patients, whose serum anti-p53 titre did not decrease after surgery, exhibited worse prognosis than patients who showed seroconversion. Thus, a correlative study between the level of tumour autoantibodies and the overall survival outcome of cancer patients (reflected in the change in tumour status or tumour burden related to the therapy) could be extremely informative for evaluating therapeutic interventions [41]. Stage-specific autoantibody biomarkers screening is thus in principle useful in predicting onset of disease, thereby providing an opportunity to intervene and delay or prevent the onset of clinical symptoms.

3.3. Immune-related adverse events

Immunotherapies have been changing the outlook for many cancer patients in recent years and immune checkpoint inhibitors represent one of several strategies now targeting the immune system for therapeutic benefits. The immune checkpoint proteins cytotoxic T-lymphocyte associated protein 4 (CTLA-4) and programmed cell death-1 (PD-1) play essential roles in central immune tolerance and are prominent targets for cancer vaccines now since inhibition of CTLA-4 and PD-1 can (re)activate the immune system to target cancer cells. Alone or in combination, clinical trials of anti-CTLA-4 and anti-PD-1 antibodies, such as Ipilimumab, Nivolumab and Pembrolizumab, have shown promising results for the treatment of melanoma, non-small cell lung-, kidney-, prostate- and head and neck cancers, as well as renal cell carcinomas, with reported therapeutic response rates approaching 70% in some cases, albeit positive immunotherapy outcomes remain cancer- and patient-specific [42].

Ipilimumab was the first anti-CTLA-4 antibody to prolong survival in patients with advanced melanoma [43, 44], with long term analysis indicating a 3-year survival of 22% across all patients with sufficient follow-up [45]. Similarly, PD-1 blockade with Nivolumab or Pembrolizumab has improved survival for metastatic melanoma, non-small cell lung cancer (NSCLC) and renal cell carcinoma (RCC) patients [46–50]. In one trial, advanced melanoma patients treated with pembrolizumab showed a response rate of 34% and a survival rate of 74% [51]. Nivolumab has been reported to result in increased response rates, survival and progression-free survival when compared to intravenous docetaxel in NSCLC [52], whilst stage III/IV melanoma patients achieved a partial tumour response, with a median progression free survival of 172 days, with only 18% experiencing grade 2 or 4 adverse events [53].

Combination check-point inhibitor treatments, targeting both CTLA-4 and PD-1, have also shown strong promise, with clinical trial data in untreated melanoma patients reporting objective response rates up to 72% (amongst patients with PD-L1-positive tumours) and with median progression-free survival of 11.5 months for ipilimumab plus nivolumab, compared to 2.9 months with ipilimumab alone and 6.9 months with nivolumab alone [54]. However, high grade immune-related adverse events (irAEs) occurred in 55% of those in the combination treatment group [54] and similarly high rates of irAEs have been reported elsewhere for anti-CTLA-4 and anti-PD-1 treatments [55].

Indeed, clinical findings on monoclonal antibody-induced adverse effects in general show that this is a wider phenomenon across different disease areas [56], which potentially compromises the effectiveness of such immunotherapies. Efforts are being channelled therefore towards predicting and monitoring undesirable immunotoxic effects and a panel of potential antibodies associated with irAE has been proposed (**Table 1**). Further exploratory studies involving autoantibody-based immunotoxicity profiling in immunotherapy patients are underway to better characterise the role and diagnostic potential of these circulating autoantibodies in irAE.

Immune-related organ involved	Antibodies
Gastro-intestinal	None
Liver	Antinuclear antibodies (ANAs)
	Anti-smooth muscle, anti-liver kidney microsomal antibody type 1, anti-liver cytosol type 1
Lung	Antinuclear antibodies (ANAs)
	Rheumatoid factor
	Anti-centromere
	Extractable nuclear antigens (ENA): anti-Sm, anti-RNP: anti-Ro (SSA)
	Anti-La (SSB): anti-Scl70, anti-Jo
Endocrine	Anti-GAD, anti-insulin, anti-carbonic anhydrase
	Anti-21 hydroxylase
	Anti-pituitary
Skin	None
Polyarthritis	Antinuclear antibodies (ANAs)
	Anti-ENA: anti-SSA, SSB, Sm
	Anti-CCP, complement fractions C3 C4 CH50
Renal	Antinuclear antibodies (ANAs)
	Complement fractions C3 CA CH50
	Anti-neutrophil cytoplasmic (ANCA)
Haematologic syndromes	Antinuclear antibodies (ANAs)
	Coombs' erythrocyte test

CCP, cyclic citrullinated peptide; GAD, glutamate decarboxylase; RNP, ribonucleoprotein; Sm, small nuclear ribonucleoprotein; SSA, Sjogren's syndrome-related antigen A; Scl, Sclerosis systemic; SSB, Sjogren's syndrome-related antigen B.

Table 1. List of proposed potential seromic autoantibodies that can be used for identifying irAEs [55].

4. Classical technological approaches to autoantibody-based biomarker discovery and validation

4.1. Western blots

Since its introduction in 1979, immunoblotting, or 'western blotting', has become a ubiquitous protein analysis technique in which proteins are separated by electrophoresis according to their molecular weight, then transferred onto a membrane before a primary antibody specific to the protein of interest is used to detect the presence and relative abundance of the target protein. Conventional western blotting allows detection of specific proteins to the level of single isotypes. However, it is associated with poor reproducibility, limited mass resolution, lack of accurate quantitation, low throughput and lengthy time to result, whilst non-specific cross-reactivity of mono- and poly-clonal primary and secondary antibodies on the blots is an everyday observation.

Certain modifications have been proposed to improve quantitation of western blots; for example, Zellner et al. reported a novel and improved quantitative Western blotting method using fluorescently labelled secondary antibodies, which extends the dynamic range of quantification and improves correlation with the protein amount [57]. Modifications based on simultaneous electrophoretic transfer of proteins from multiple strips of polyacrylamide gels to a single membrane sheet have also been reported to increase the data output per single blotting cycle by up to 10-fold [58], whilst resulting in reduced immunoblotting-derived signal errors and improving the overall data accuracy [58]. However, in the context of biomarker discovery, western blotting is typically only used as a validation method rather than as a primary method of identifying biomarkers.

4.2. Enzyme-linked immunosorbent assay (ELISA)

ELISA, unlike western blotting, is adaptable to higher throughput of samples as it is typically performed in 96-well microtitre plates whereby plate handling and detection systems can be automated. ELISA can be used to determine the exact amount of a specific protein in a sample, making it more readily quantitative as a technique compared to western blotting. The signals are usually produced by chromogenic reaction that generate a coloured product, which is quantified by spectrophotometry. There are four types of ELISA – sandwich, direct, indirect and competitive – which essentially differ in whether the antigen or a capture antibody is immobilised onto the surface (**Figure 3**).

In the context of autoantibody detection, the direct and indirect ELISA formats are most commonly used, but are better suited to the analysis of a larger number of samples against a small number of antigens in screening, verification and validation applications rather than as a primary discovery platform [59]. Furthermore, standard ELISA often has relatively low sensitivity and detection usually depends on enzymatic amplification of signal at the end of the assay. In addition, ELISA can also give false positives due to cross-reactivity of the detecting antibodies with other proteins in the sample. As sensitivity and specificity are prerequisites of any biomarker discovery platform, traditional ELISA may not be the ideal choice when it comes to identifying biologically relevant and meaningful disease biomarkers.

4.3. Mass spectrometry

The use of mass spectrometry for serum biomarker discovery is in theory straightforward since results are obtained in the form of identified and quantified proteins that are then compared between pathological and control groups [60]. Recent advances in mass spectrometry

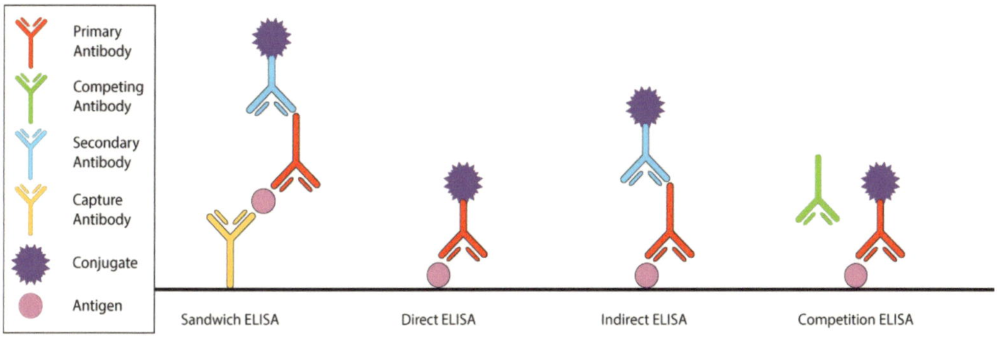

Figure 3. Types of ELISA assays.

instrumentation have significantly improved the depth, breadth and reproducibility of protein identifications in many biological samples, which in turn has aided the identification of meaningful signatures that have diagnostic potential. However, whilst mass spectrometry is in general a powerful approach for unbiased biomarker identification, there are some limitations, particularly in serum biomarker discovery, due to the complex nature of serum and its wide dynamic range of protein concentrations (spanning 12-orders of magnitude), as well as to the intrinsic mass spectrometry sensitivity (>μg/mL) in detecting analytes which usually range between 50 pg/mL and 10 ng/mL in serum [60]. Furthermore, mass spectrometry-based proteomics remains heavily constrained today in its ability to differentiate and assign function to individual antibody sequences within a large collection of immunoglobulins: this is partly because the affinity-matured antibody sequences are not germ-line encoded (and therefore do not appear in the proteome databases that underpin tandem mass spectrometry-based protein identifications) and is partly because both light and heavy chains are required for antigen specificity in an immunoglobulin, yet that pairing between light and heavy chain sequences (as well as the connectivity between the complementary determining regions with each light and heavy chain) is lost during proteolytic digest before mass spectrometry analysis; moreover, antigen specificity cannot yet be predicted *de novo* from the primary immunoglobulin sequence. As a result, mass spectrometry is currently not well suited to the challenge of autoantibody biomarker discovery [61]; alternative technological platforms are therefore required to unravel the complexity of the human immunoglobulin repertoire and to detect and quantify novel autoantibody/autoantigen pairs in biological samples.

4.4. Serologic proteome analysis

Serologic Proteome Analysis (SERPA) is a classical immunoproteomics approach to autoantigen discovery that provides a robust way of screening antibody reactivity profiles in sera from patients with various diseases. The method – which is essentially an adaption of western blotting - involves separating proteins from a biological sample (e.g. a tissue homogenate or cell lysate) using 2-dimensional electrophoresis on large format gels and then immunoblotting with patient or control sera. Unique protein spots identified by following blotting with patient but not control sera are excised from the gels and identified by mass spectrometry. However, the inherently high gel-to-gel variability and relatively low resolving power of individual gels impacts on the accuracy of spot picking and imposes a limitation due to co-migrating proteins, which is especially problematic for low-abundance protein targets. Several modifications have been suggested to address such limitations, including multi-colour fluorescence-based 2-D gel immunoproteomics approaches [62], but these still do not address the fundamental issues of the limited resolving power of the gels, the modest limit of detection or the throughput for SERPA. This technology is thus less widely used for autoantigen discovery now and has been largely supplanted by newer technologies that are better able to overcome these limitations.

4.5. Serological analysis of recombinant cDNA expression libraries (SEREX)

SEREX is one of the oldest methods for autoantigen discovery and utilises human cDNA expression libraries to profile autoantibody repertoires. The methodology for SEREX initially involves generation of a cDNA library from a cancer tissue or tumour cell line, followed by cloning of that library into a suitable expression vector, clonal separation of the library and expression of the encoded proteins in *Escherichia coli* cells grown on solid media. Colonies are then transferred to a nitrocellulose or PVDF membrane, lysed and the expressed recombinant proteins blotted with sera from patients and healthy controls. Sero-reactive proteins are then identified by sequencing the cDNA from positive colonies [63], which makes it more sensitive than the SERPA method since the latter relies on direct protein identification and is therefore limited by absolute protein abundance. Furthermore, the clonal separation of the members of the cDNA expression library provides greater resolving power than the gel-based SERPA method. However, as with all library-based screening methods, over-sampling is required to ensure that all members of the library are examined in SEREX: thus, if for example the cDNA library contains 10^4 unique clones, then at least 10^5 colonies would need to be screened for complete coverage, so even with the advent of colony picking and arraying robots, SEREX remains a relatively low throughput method.

The first cancer testis antigen, NY-ESO-1, was identified by SEREX by analysing tumour associated antigens (TAAs) that elicited a high titre IgG antibody in sera from patients with different types of cancer [64]. SEREX has also been successfully used to identify several TAAs that generate a humoral immune response in cancers such as those from the kidney, lung, breast and colon [63]. However, a fundamental limitation of SEREX is that the method lacks the ability to differentiate or detect post-translational modifications (PTMs) that are likely to play a significant role in autoimmune diseases [62] and cancers [63]. This approach also restricts the types of TAAs identified to those that can be expressed in a prokaryotic system and also effectively excludes TAAs that require folding mechanisms unique to eukaryotes to achieve the correct conformational epitope for recognition [63]. SEREX may also miss TAAs that are represented by truncated cDNAs in the library, since the encoded protein may lack specific epitopes or even whole domains. Furthermore, identification of TAAs is inherently limited to those that were expressed by the specific patient tumour or cell line from which the cDNA library was derived, which means that more than one cDNA library may be required to identify comprehensive set of TAAs for different cancers [63]. In addition, the presence of the crude prokaryotic cell lysate in every spot can give rise to high background binding in SEREX assays. Thus, for many of these reasons, SEREX has largely been superseded now by protein microarray technologies that are based on purified recombinant proteins.

5. Protein microarrays

Protein microarrays are a versatile, miniaturised platform used to simultaneously characterise the biomolecular interactions of thousands of different proteins that are spotted in defined locations on a solid support; as such, protein microarrays represent a natural technological evolution from ELISA, SERPA and SEREX. Protein microarrays in principle allow the quantitative analysis of binding of a wide variety of analytes - including antibodies, proteins, DNA, RNA, small molecules, lipids, enzymes as well as peptides - to the arrayed proteins. The three types of protein microarrays that are commonly used are analytical, functional and reverse-phase microarrays. Analytical protein arrays, or antibody arrays, are ideal for quantification of different known proteins in a biological sample, monitoring protein expression levels and protein profiling in what amounts to miniaturised, highly multiplexed ELISA assays. Functional protein microarrays can be sub-divided into those based on recombinant proteins and those based on native proteins and can be used for autoantibody and immune response profiling, biomolecular interaction profiling and identification of enzyme substrates, amongst others [1]. Reverse-phase protein arrays are comprised of spots of different crude tissue homogenates or cell lysates and are suited for detection of known proteins in multiple tissues/cells based on blotting of the reverse-phase arrays with antigen-specific antibodies. In general, protein microarrays can be applied in diagnostic and therapeutic research, through new biomarker discovery for disease staging and monitoring, potential drug-target evaluation and for identification of new drug targets. Of the different protein array types, functional protein arrays appear best suited to autoantigen discovery and autoantibody profiling and are discussed in more detail below.

5.1. Recombinant protein production

Different protein production systems can be employed to produce recombinant proteins in sufficient quantities for protein microarray fabrication. The key problem associated with recombinant protein production is identifying the best expression system for a particular protein. To date, there is no universally applicable protein expression system [65]. Each system has its advantages and disadvantages; therefore, the choice of expression system selection should be based on the properties of the recombinant protein as well as the scale of expression required. Although exploring multiple expression systems in parallel sounds enticing, factors such as protein solubility, yield, speed and cost need to be taken into consideration as it involves substantial resources. Choosing the right system for protein expression can be particularly important in obtaining biologically active and functional recombinant proteins [1].

Bacteria, notably *E. coli*, represent the most commonly used expression systems for protein production since they give high protein yields at a relatively low cost, require simple and rapid culture conditions, and are highly scalable. In addition, many parameters can be altered to optimise expression levels of protein. However, inefficient disulfide bond formation, insolubility, aggregation and poor folding of proteins have been reported using this method, as well as very minimal capability in performing post-translational modifications [65].

Expression of proteins in yeast is a common alternative to prokaryotic expression systems as it is a well-defined and economical eukaryotic expression system. Commonly used yeast strains include *Saccharomyces cerevisiae* and *Pichia pastoris,* although other yeast strains have also been reported. Proteins expressed using both strains fold efficiently and numerous post-translational modifications can occur; *P. pastoris* typically gives better protein yields than *S. cerevisiae* [65]. However, a major disadvantage of the yeast expression systems is that they do not mimic protein glycosylation patterns from mammalian cells, with proteins tending to be hyperglycosylated due to the presence of large mannose glycans. Furthermore, lysis conditions for yeast are typically harsh and induce many endogenous proteases, meaning that the extracted recombinant proteins are often significantly proteolysed.

Baculoviruses belong to a diverse group of large double-stranded DNA viruses that infect many different species of insects as their natural hosts but are highly species-specific and are not known to propagate in any non-invertebrate host. Baculoviral expression systems yield good expression levels, especially for intracellular proteins, and typically produce functionally active, recombinant mammalian proteins that are properly folded and oligomerised and which contain correct disulfide bonds, as well as mammalian-like post-translational modifications, including glycosylation, so are both structurally and functionally similar to their native counterparts [65].

Mammalian expression systems are preferred by some researchers as they produce more 'humanised' proteins, with the most biologically-relevant post-translational modifications and native folding. Amongst the most widely used mammalian cells include HeLa, human embryonic kidney-derived (HEK293) epithelial cells, Chinese hamster ovary cells (CHOs) and African green monkey kidney cells (COS). However, mammalian protein expression systems require more demanding culture conditions compared to other systems [65] so are significantly more challenging for high throughput expression purposes.

5.2. Surface chemistry

The microarray surface chemistry plays a critical role in determining protein microarray quality. Slide surfaces vary: aldehyde and epoxy-derivatized glass surfaces are used for random attachment through amines, whereas nitrocellulose, hydrogel or metal surfaces for attachment of affinity-purified proteins. An ideal surface chemistry should resist nonspecific adsorption, whilst preserving the folded structure of the arrayed proteins [1].

Common challenges associated with slide surface chemistry include high background and incorrect protein orientation or conformation of proteins, whereby all functional binding sites are not readily available for interaction. Proteins have various hydrophobic domains and charged patches, so tend to adsorb non-specifically to most solid surfaces resulting in the disruption of protein 3-D structure and eventually complete loss of activity. This indirectly gives rise to the second issue - the loss of protein conformation upon immobilisation. In particular, when the functional domains interact excessively with a solid surface, the orientation of the proteins may be altered or completely lost, resulting in the subsequent disruption of the functional domains and loss of discontinuous epitopes [66]. Partial or complete denaturation of proteins on the arrayed surface is also deleterious for downstream autoantibody binding since it is well known that antibodies tend to bind non-specifically to exposed hydrophobic epitopes, giving rise to false positive signals in autoantibody profiling assays.

Proteins can be immobilised onto a microarray surface via encapsulation, surface adsorption, covalent attachment or affinity binding (**Figure 4**), which are further described below [67].

Encapsulation of a purified protein on a solid surface involves suspending the protein in a random orientation within a 3D gel pad (e.g. acrylamide or agarose) on an array surface; this approach provides a high capacity for immobilisation and thereby enhances the sensitivity of subsequent assays. A drawback of the technique, however, is that the size of the protein or other ligand applied may restrict diffusion into the gel, resulting in stronger signals at the periphery of the gel pad. This challenge may be surmounted when using different cross-linkers that can improve the porosity of the gel pads [68].

Immobilisation of purified proteins via noncovalent adsorption is a straightforward, reversible method that involves protein attachment onto a solid support through weak, non-specific interactions, including van der Waals hydrophobic interactions and electrostatic interactions. Commonly used surfaces here include nitrocellulose-coated and amine-terminated glass slides. Although this approach can provide high protein loading onto the surface, the orientation of the immobilised protein cannot be controlled, resulting in variable reaction efficiency, accuracy and reproducibility of the resultant arrays [69]. Furthermore, the underlying surfaces tend to be relatively denaturing towards the arrayed proteins [1].

Covalent attachment takes place by chemically cross-linking proteins to the surface through the nucleophilic residues lysine or cysteine. These residues are cross-linked to surface-bound ligands that are terminated with aldehyde, epoxy, or N-hydroxysuccinamide moieties. Irreversible immobilisation of a wide range of proteins to the carrier surfaces are feasible using covalent attachment, but the non-specific modification of surface residues on the arrayed protein carries the risk of altering the activity and folded structure of those proteins [70].

Affinity capture is a particularly advantageous way to immobilise proteins, since it circumvents many of the limitations of other approaches described above. Typical affinity capture methods include use of biotinylated, hexa-His-tagged, glutathione S transferase tagged or Halo tagged recombinant proteins [1], with orientation of the immobilised protein being controlled via the tag, thereby aiding in preserving the structure and function of the arrayed proteins.

Numerous human protein microarray platforms are available today for autoantibody research, including Immunome arrays (Sengenics, Singapore), Nucleic Acid Programmable Arrays (BioDesign Institute, Arizona), Human Protein Atlas Protein Fragment Arrays (SciLifeLab, Sweden), HuProt arrays (CDI Laboratories, USA) and ProtoArrays (ThermoFischer, USA). These various human protein microarray platforms have differing protein content and make

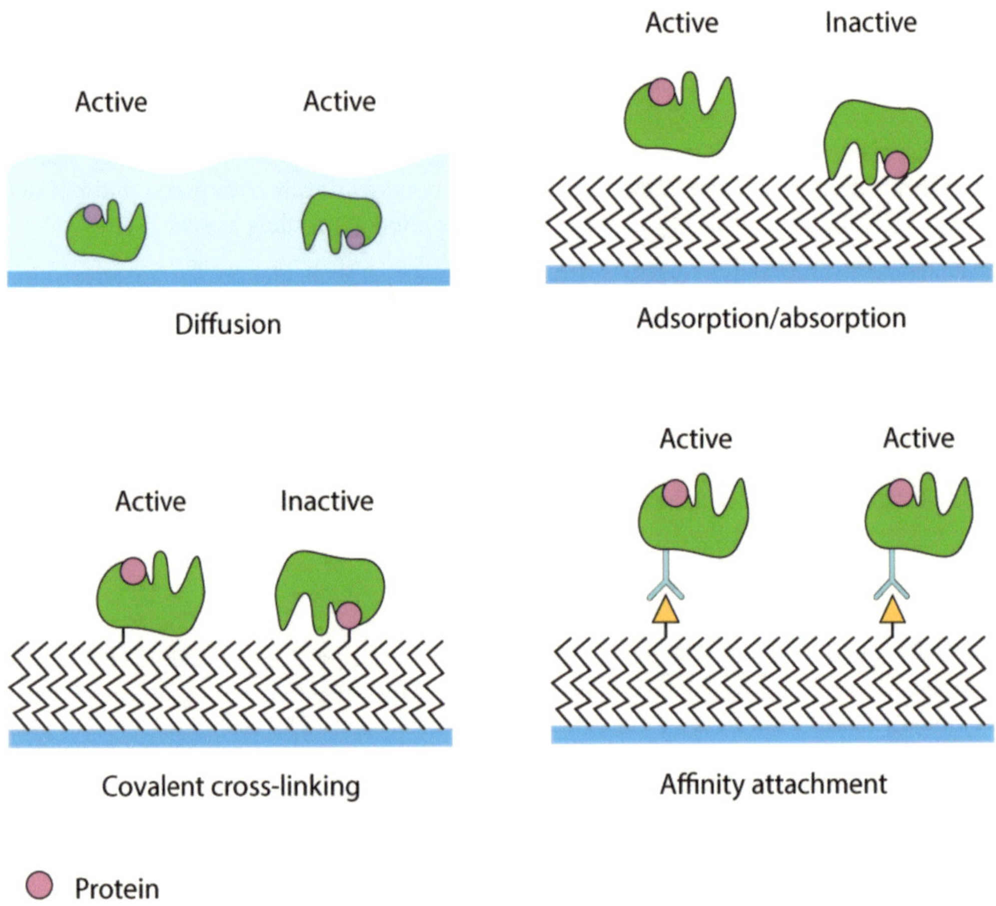

Figure 4. Various methods of protein immobilisation onto a solid support; encapsulation, surface adsorption, covalent cross-linking and affinity attachment.

different use of the various protein expression systems, surface chemistries and immobilisation strategies described above, all of which gives rise to differences in technical performance, as has been reviewed recently [1].

By way of example, proteins on the Immunome array are expressed in a baculoviral system as in-frame fusions to a biotin carboxyl carrier protein (BCCP) folding marker, that itself becomes biotinylated *in vivo* or *in vitro* only when the fusion protein is correctly folded. Immunome's surface chemistry is based on a hydrogel polymer that dramatically reduces non-specific background binding to the array surface whilst providing an aqueous-like environment for the arrayed proteins. The hydrogel matrix is derivatised with a low density of streptavidin molecules that are held away from the underlying array substrate, providing a selective surface for binding of biotinylated proteins (**Figure 5**). This helps to ensure that each protein immobilised on the array retains its native conformation, correctly folding and functionality on the array surface.

5.3. Sensitivity and reproducibility

Quantification of autoantibody biomarkers using a protein microarray starts with the production of recombinant proteins, printing of the proteins onto a solid support, probing them with serum or plasma samples and finally capturing interactions using fluorescent-labelled secondary antibodies. Protein microarrays have thus often been referred to as miniaturised version of ELISA. Miniaturisation allows a high overall sensitivity as analyte measurement is conducted while retaining the highest concentration per unit volume attainable for the given sample, with decreased reaction times due to short diffusion distances [71]. Furthermore, fluorescent-based signal detection in protein microarrays offers lower limits of detection (as low as 1 pg/mL; [72]) and greater dynamic range (up to 5 orders of magnitude; [73]) than colourimetric readouts in typical ELISAs. In addition to their greater sensitivity compared to ELISA, protein arrays are also superior in terms of multiplexing, as thousands of proteins can be printed onto glass slides in replicates and analysed simultaneously.

Given the capacity for multiplexing, as well as the high-throughput, low sample consumption, remarkable sensitivity and reproducibility of protein arrays, this platform is rapidly proving now to be very well suited to the challenges of autoantibody biomarker discovery. However, when choosing the optimal platform for discovery research, important factors such as the protein expression system used and the surface chemistry of the platform should be considered carefully to ensure that only biologically-meaningful autoantibody biomarkers that have the potential to be translated into clinical use will be discovered.

5.4. Protein microarray-based autoantibody discovery

Microarrays fabricated with proteins derived from tissues or cell-line, or recombinant proteins have been used in many studies to identify potential autoantibody biomarkers for cancer, a few examples of which follow.

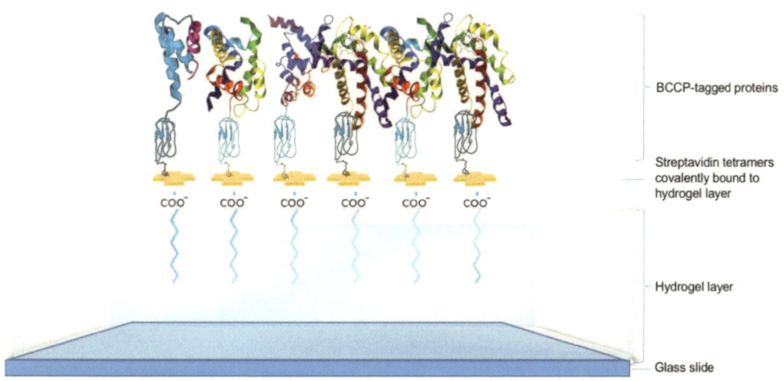

Figure 5. Depiction of the slide surface chemistry of the immunome protein array. Individually-purified BCCP-tagged proteins are immobilised onto customised hydrogel-coated surfaces such that they retain folded structure and function in an aqueous environment and behave as if they are in free solution.

Native protein microarrays: Nam et al. demonstrated the feasibility of manufacturing a native protein microarray using chromatographic techniques and microarray printing technology. Here, a crude cell lysate was resolved in 2 dimensions using liquid-based isoelectric focusing followed by reverse-phase liquid chromatography, resulting in 1760 fractions which were then printed on a nitrocellulose surface and used to screen sera from cancer patients vs. healthy controls to identify fractions containing cancer-specific reactive autoantigens. Fractions corresponding to reactive spots were analysed using mass spectrometry to identify cancer-specific autoantigens, which revealed that 9/15 colon cancer patients, but neither of the healthy controls, produced autoantibodies against ubiquitin C-terminal hydrolase isozyme (UCH-L3). Autoantibody production against UCH-L3 was confirmed by Western blot in 19 of 43 (44%) additional colon cancer patients [74].

Antibody microarrays: in order to identify prostate cancer-associated autoantibodies, well-characterised monoclonal antibodies were arrayed onto nanoparticle slides to capture native antigens from prostate cancer cells, which were subsequently incubated with fluorescently-labelled IgG from patients with prostate cancer and benign prostate hyperplasia (BPH). The study revealed that prostate cancer patients had higher autoantibody levels against TLN1, TARDBP, LEDGF, CALD1, and PARK7 when compared to patients with BPH. The study concluded that PSA alone produced sensitivity- and specificity-values of 12.2 and 80%, respectively, whereas the collective panel produced sensitivity- and specificity-values of 95 and 80%, respectively [75].

Functional protein microarrays: a cancer antigen microarray, comprising 123 full length, folded, recombinant tumour-associated antigens expressed in insect cells was used to identify autoantibodies that differentiate prostate cancer patients from benign prostatic hyperplasia (BPH) and other disease controls. The study identified 41 potential diagnostic/therapeutic antigen biomarkers for prostate cancer and found that autoantibody titres against GAGE1, ROPN1, SPANX1 and PRKCZ were high in prostate cancer patients, whereas autoantibody titres against MAGEB1 and PRKCZ were higher in BPH controls. Of the 41 potential antigens identified, FGFR2, COL6A1 and CALM1 were identified in urine from the same patients by shotgun proteomics [76].

Functional protein microarrays have also been used to identify autoantibodies against autoantigens in a number of other infectious or autoimmune-related diseases, including malaria and Parkinson's disease (PD). In malaria, *Plasmodium knowlesi* infection results in an autoimmune-like response in some individuals that has been hypothesised to play a protective role against malarial infection. Using the Sengenics Immunome protein array comprising 1636 correctly folded human antigens, 24 antigens with high reactivity to serum autoantibodies were identified, which may serve as potential biomarkers for asymptomatic malaria, mild malaria, or predictive biomarkers for severe malaria [77].

PD is a chronic and progressive neurodegenerative disorder, and a positive correlation is associated with *Helicobacter pylori* (*H. pylori*) and PD motor severity. The Sengenics Immunome protein array was used to screen *H. pylori*-seropositive PD patients and *H. pylori*-seronegative PD patients in a study that identified 13 significant autoantibodies, of which 8 were up-regulated and 5 down-regulated in the case group. Identified autoantigens included Nuclear factor I subtype A (NFIA), Platelet-derived growth factor B (PDGFB) and Eukaryotic translation initiation factor 4A3 (elFA3) [78].

Other protein microarray platforms, including nucleic acid programmable protein arrays (NAPPA), HuProt arrays, Protoarrays and Human Protein Atlas Protein Fragment Arrays, have also found utility in autoantibody biomarker discovery applications across a wide variety of disease areas, including a broad spectrum of cancers and autoimmune diseases, as well as several neurological disorders and inflammatory disorders, as recently reviewed elsewhere [1].

6. Biomarker validation

Biomarkers can be used for variety of purposes including disease prediction, diagnosis and treatment monitoring. However, while there are thousands of papers reporting discovery of potential biomarkers, very few of these have been validated and approved by the Food and Drug Administration (FDA) for clinical use (**Table 2**), despite preliminary reports of good sensitivity and specificity. This highlights the reality that biomarker validation is a challenging process with multiple criteria that need to be fulfilled before the markers can be approved use in clinical settings. There are also multiple stages where attrition can occur in the validation process, including poor study design, variations in sample collection, and the simple failure of the biomarkers in blinded validations, as discussed further below:

A key requirement for all biomarker validation is that the biomarker demonstrates a correlation with specific pathophysiological processes or serves as a surrogate endpoint in a clinical trial. Diagnostic precision and accuracy are key technical parameters, since inaccurate or variable results, as well as false positive and false negative results, could lead to misdiagnosis that could bring about unwanted sequelae.

Typical biomarker discovery programs are initially set up as case–control studies, with clearly defined and well-separated clinical groups. However, in real world settings, the diagnostic challenge is often not to distinguish diseased from healthy, but to differentiate amongst people with similar clinical symptoms but different underlying disorders. As a first step towards validation therefore, once candidate biomarkers have been identified from an initial discovery study, a scientifically sound and statistically-powered validation cohort needs to be designed to test the diagnostic power of the biomarkers in the context of 'diseased patients' and 'other disease' controls. Power calculations are used to determine the sample size required to identify reproducible, precise and accurate biomarkers that qualify for clinical utilisation and this cohort is then typically sub-divided into a training cohort and a larger blinded validation cohort. Typically, the clinical sensitivity and specificity of a larger set of candidate biomarkers from the discovery research is first assessed in the training cohort and the best performing markers that survive are taken forward for further evaluation in the blinded validation cohort.

Biomarker	Cancer type	Clinical use	Specimen
Pro2PSA	Prostate	Discriminating cancer from benign disease	Serum
Free PSA	Prostate	Discriminating cancer from benign disease	
Total PSA	Prostate	Prostate cancer diagnosis and monitoring	
ROMA (HE4 + CA-125)	Ovarian	Prediction of malignancy	
OVA1 (multiple proteins)	Ovarian	Prediction of malignancy	
HE4	Ovarian	Monitoring recurrence or progression of disease	
Fibrin/fibrinogen degradation product (DR-70)	Colorectal	Monitoring progression of disease	
AFP-L3%	Hepatocellular	Risk assessment for development of disease	
CA27.29	Breast	Monitoring disease response to therapy	
CA15–3	Breast	Monitoring disease response to therapy	Serum, plasma
CA19–9	Pancreatic	Monitoring disease status	
CA-125	Ovarian	Monitoring disease progression, response to therapy	
Thyroglobulin	Thyroid	Aid in monitoring	
Alpha-fetoprotein (AFP)	Testicular	Management of cancer	
Carcinoembryonic antigen	Not specified	Aid in management and prognosis	
p63 protein	Prostate	Aid in differential diagnosis	FFPE tissue
c-Kit	Gastrointestinal stromal tumours	Detection of tumours, aid in selection of patients	
Oestrogen receptor (ER)	Breast	Prognosis, response to therapy	
Progesterone receptor (PR)	Breast	Prognosis, response to therapy	
Her-2/neu	Breast	Assessment for therapy	
Circulating tumour cells (EpCAM, CD45, cytokeratins 8, 18+, 19+)	Breast	Prediction of cancer progression and survival	Whole blood
Nuclear Mitotic Apparatus protein (NuMA, NMP22)	Bladder	Diagnosis and monitoring of disease (professional and home use)	Urine
Alpha-fetoprotein (AFP)	Testicular	Management of cancer	Amniotic fluid
Human haemoglobin (faecal occult blood)	Colorectal	Detection of faecal occult blood (home use)	Faeces

Table 2. List of FDA-approved tumour markers commonly used in clinical practice which mainly consist of serum and plasma biomarkers.

Statistically-powered validation cohorts often run into hundreds of patients, so obtaining quality serum or plasma samples in sufficient quantities from a disease cohort, as well as from matched healthy and other disease controls, can therefore sometimes be a challenge. Furthermore, biomarker validation is a complex and lengthy process, meaning that the validation assay methods themselves need to be rapid, robust, reproducible, inexpensive and easy to setup and run, potentially in different laboratories.

Even after considering the aforementioned factors, it often turns out that the candidate biomarker is simply not robust, sensitive or specific enough to penetrate into a clinical setting. Ideal candidates for multiplexed panels would be markers whose qualitative and/or quantitative expression is unique to the disease. However, particularly in the case of cancers, identifying truly disease specific markers has proved problematic; for example, MAGE-A3 was originally thought to be 'tumour specific' marker but was later found to be detectable in healthy tissues as well [71]. It is therefore not surprising that biomarkers with early diagnostic potential initially obtained in studies conducted in laboratory settings can often not be confirmed in later clinical validation and screening settings, resulting in high attrition rates during biomarker validation.

7. Conclusion

Autoantibodies have gained considerable attention in the medical diagnostic field as candidate diagnostic and prognostic biomarkers in many different disease areas, since they are in theory detectable many years before clinical symptoms appear. This particular property of autoantibodies makes them attractive tools for early diagnosis of disease. However, identification and validation of autoantibody biomarkers has historically been constrained by the available technological approaches and the high attrition rates during studies on larger cohorts.

To increase the success rate in biomarker discovery and validation, the correct technique as well as the right number of samples and analytes to be used for each phase should be carefully planned and designed as depicted in **Figure 6**. The current gold standard for biomarker validation remains ELISA, which is regularly utilised for confirmatory studies as it allows a relatively high-throughput of samples and is a versatile and robust tool. Thus, protein microarray analysis is often compared against the quantitative data of ELISA assays [79]. However, ELISAs routinely permit only single antigen detection per well and often require relatively large volumes of samples compared to other more miniaturised, high-throughput methods. This leaves substantial scope for protein microarrays to be used in both the discovery and validation of panels of autoantibody biomarkers, since they represent a sensitive, highly reproducible, multiplexed and high throughput experimental platform for autoantibody quantitation; this will undoubtedly be aided by the underlying protein microarray platforms themselves gaining regulatory approval for use as clinical diagnostics.

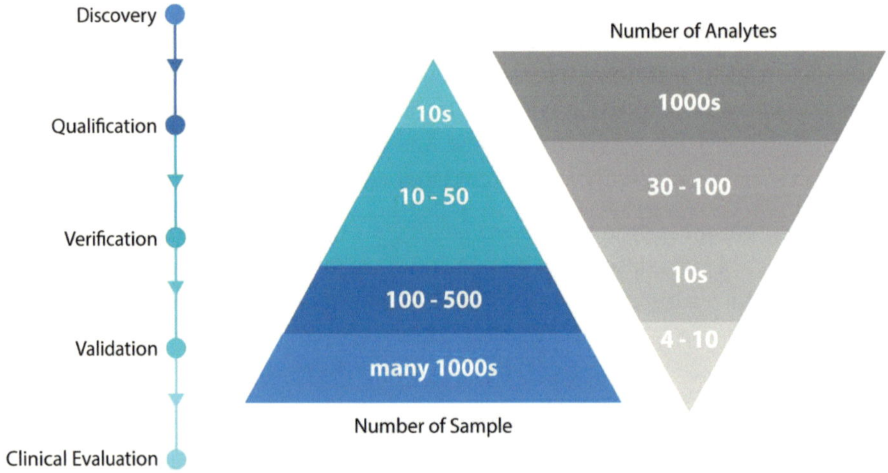

Figure 6. Phases of biomarker discovery pipeline. Each phase requires different technologies and study design.

Author details

Farhanah Aziz[1], Muneera Smith[2] and Jonathan M Blackburn[1,2]*

*Address all correspondence to: jonathan.blackburn@uct.ac.za

1 Sengenics Corporation, Singapore

2 Institute of Infectious Disease and Molecular Medicine, Department of Integrative Biomedical Sciences, Faculty of Health Sciences, University of Cape Town, Cape Town, South Africa

References

[1] Duarte JG, Blackburn JM. Advances in the development of human protein microarrays. Expert Review of Proteomics. Jul. 2017;**14**(7):627-641

[2] Schroeder HW, Cavacini L. Structure and function of immunoglobulins. The Journal of Allergy and Clinical Immunology. Feb. 2010;**125**(2):S41-S52

[3] Moder KG, Wener MH, Weisman MH, Ishimori ML, Wallace DJ, Buckeridge DL, et al. Measurement of antinuclear antibodies by multiplex immunoassay: A prospective, multi-center clinical evaluation. Journal of Rheumatol. 2007 May;**34**(5):978-986

[4] Ma W-T, Chang C, Gershwin ME, Lian Z-X. Development of autoantibodies precedes clinical manifestations of autoimmune diseases: A comprehensive review. Journal of Autoimmunity. Sep. 2017;**83**:95-112

[5] Wardemann H, Nussenzweig MC. B-cell self-tolerance in humans. Advances in Immunology. 2007;**95**:83-110

[6] Kim H-J, Verbinnen B, Tang X, Lu L, Cantor H. Inhibition of follicular T-helper cells by CD8+ regulatory T cells is essential for self tolerance. Nature. Sep. 2010;**467**(7313):328-332

[7] Carl PL, Temple BR, Cohen PL. Most nuclear systemic autoantigens are extremely disordered proteins: Implications for the etiology of systemic autoimmunity. Arthritis Research & Therapy. 2005;**7**(6):1360-1374

[8] Alvarez Arias DA et al. Disruption of CD8+ Treg activity results in expansion of T follicular helper cells and enhanced antitumor immunity. Cancer Immunology Research. Mar. 2014;**2**(3):207-216

[9] Elkon K, Casali P. Nature and functions of autoantibodies. Nature Clinical Practice. Rheumatology. Sep. 2008;**4**(9):491-498

[10] Burska AN et al. Autoantibodies to posttranslational modifications in rheumatoid arthritis. Mediators of Inflammation. 2014;**2014**:1-19

[11] Kaveri SV, Silverman GJ, Bayry J. Natural IgM in immune equilibrium and harnessing their therapeutic potential. Journal of Immunology. Feb. 2012;**188**(3):939-945

[12] Grönwall C, Vas J, Silverman GJ. Protective roles of natural IgM antibodies. Frontiers in Immunology. 2012;**3**:1-10

[13] Ceccarelli F et al. Genetic factors in systemic lupus Erythematosus: Contribution to disease phenotype. Journal of Immunology Research. 2015;**2015**:1-11

[14] Förster M et al. Genetic control of antibody production during collagen-induced arthritis development in heterogeneous stock mice. Arthritis and Rheumatism. Nov. 2012;**64**(11):3594-3603

[15] Álvarez-Cermeño JC, Villar LM. Multiple sclerosis: Genetic variability affects CNS IgG production in MS. Nature Reviews. Neurology. Jun. 2015;**11**(6):313-314

[16] Poletaev A, Boura P. The immune system, natural autoantibodies and general homeostasis in health and disease. Hippokratia. Oct. 2011;**15**(4):295-298

[17] Merbl Y, Zucker-Toledano M, Quintana FJ, Cohen IR. Newborn humans manifest autoantibodies to defined self molecules detected by antigen microarray informatics. The Journal of Clinical Investigation. Mar. 2007;**117**(3):712-718

[18] Madi A et al. Organization of the autoantibody repertoire in healthy newborns and adults revealed by system level informatics of antigen microarray data. Proceedings of the National Academy of Sciences of the United States of America. Aug. 2009;**106**(34): 14484-14489

[19] Klein SL, Flanagan KL. Sex differences in immune responses. Nature Reviews. Immunology. Oct. 2016;**16**(10):626-638

[20] Khan D, Ansar Ahmed S. The immune system is a natural target for estrogen action: Opposing effects of Estrogen in two prototypical autoimmune diseases. Frontiers in Immunology. 2015;**6**:1-8

[21] Rahat MA, Shakya J. Parallel aspects of the microenvironment in cancer and autoimmune disease. Mediators of Inflammation. 2016;**2016**:1-17

[22] Watson S. Autoimmune Diseases: Types, Symptoms, Causes and More. Healthline Media; Oct-2017

[23] Sulzer D et al. T cells from patients with Parkinson's disease recognize α-synuclein peptides. Nature. Jun. 2017;**546**(7660):656-661

[24] Brudek T et al. Autoimmune antibody decline in Parkinson's disease and multiple system atrophy; a step towards immunotherapeutic strategies. Molecular Neurodegeneration. 2017;**12**(1):44

[25] Landhuis E. Obscure Disease May Offer Backdoor to New Treatments for Alzheimer's and Other Killers. Scientific American; 2016. Available from: https://www.scientificamerican.com/article/obscure-disease-may-offer-backdoor-to-new-treatments-for-alzheimer-s-and-other-killers/

[26] Sevigny J et al. The antibody aducanumab reduces Aβ plaques in Alzheimer's disease. Nature. 2016;**537**(7618):50-56

[27] Theander E, Jonsson R, Sjöström B, Brokstad K, Olsson P, Henriksson G. Prediction of Sjögren's syndrome years before diagnosis and identification of patients with early onset and severe disease course by autoantibody profiling. Arthritis & Rheumatology (Hoboken, N.J.). Sep. 2015;**67**(9):2427-2436

[28] Taylor P, Gartemann J, Hsieh J, Creeden J. A systematic review of serum biomarkers anti-cyclic citrullinated peptide and rheumatoid factor as tests for rheumatoid arthritis. Autoimmune Diseases. 2011;**2011**:1-18

[29] Wu J, Li L. Autoantibodies in Alzheimer's disease: Potential biomarkers, pathogenic roles, and therapeutic implications. Journal of Biomedical Research. Sep. 2016

[30] Davydova TV, Voskresenskaya NI, Fomina VG, Vetrile LA, Doronina OA. Induction of autoantibodies to glutamate in patients with Alzheimer's disease. Bulletin of Experimental Biology and Medicine. Feb. 2007;**143**(2):182-183

[31] Boyle P et al. Clinical validation of an autoantibody test for lung cancer. Annals of Oncology. Feb. 2011;**22**(2):383-389

[32] Wang X et al. Autoantibody signatures in prostate cancer. The New England Journal of Medicine. Sep. 2005;**353**(12):1224-1235

[33] Chatterjee M et al. Diagnostic markers of ovarian cancer by high-throughput antigen cloning and detection on arrays. Cancer Research. Jan. 2006;**66**(2):1181-1190

[34] DeMarshall C et al. Utility of autoantibodies as biomarkers for diagnosis and staging of neurodegenerative diseases. International Review of Neurobiology. 2015;**122**:1-51

[35] Zaenker P, Ziman MR. Serologic autoantibodies as diagnostic cancer biomarkers--a review. Cancer Epidemiology, Biomarkers & Prevention. Dec. 2013;**22**(12):2161-2181

[36] Kita T et al. Extracellular cAMP-dependent protein kinase (ECPKA) in melanoma. Cancer Letters. May 2004;**208**(2):187-191

[37] Xie C et al. A novel multiplex assay combining autoantibodies plus PSA has potential implications for classification of prostate cancer from non-malignant cases. Journal of Translational Medicine. Apr. 2011;**9**:1-11

[38] Chapman C et al. Autoantibodies in breast cancer: Their use as an aid to early diagnosis. Annals of Oncology. May 2007;**18**(5):868-873

[39] Insel RA et al. Staging presymptomatic type 1 diabetes: A scientific statement of JDRF, the Endocrine Society, and the American Diabetes Association. Diabetes Care. Oct. 2015;**38**(10):1964-1974

[40] Cai H-YY, Wang X-HH, Tian Y, Gao L-YY, Zhang L-JJ, Zhang Z-YY. Changes of serum p53 antibodies and clinical significance of radiotherapy for esophageal squamous cell carcinoma. World Journal of Gastroenterology. Jul. 2008;**14**(25):4082-4086

[41] Shimada H et al. Perioperative changes of serum p53 antibody titer is a predictor for survival in patients with esophageal squamous cell carcinoma. World Journal of Surgery. Feb. 2009;**33**(2):272-277

[42] Swart M, Verbrugge I, Beltman JB. Combination approaches with immune-checkpoint blockade in cancer therapy. Frontiers in Oncology. Nov. 2016;**6**:1-16

[43] Hodi FS et al. Improved survival with ipilimumab in patients with metastatic melanoma. The New England Journal of Medicine. 2010;**363**(8):711-723

[44] Robert C et al. Ipilimumab plus Dacarbazine for previously untreated metastatic melanoma. The New England Journal of Medicine. 2011;**364**(26):2517-2526

[45] Schadendorf D et al. Pooled analysis of long-term survival data from phase II and phase III trials of Ipilimumab in Unresectable or metastatic melanoma. Journal of Clinical Oncology. 2015;**33**(17):1889-1894

[46] Herbst RS et al. Predictive correlates of response to the anti-PD-L1 antibody MPDL3280A in cancer patients. Nature. Nov. 2014;**515**(7528):563-567

[47] Garon EB et al. Pembrolizumab for the treatment of non-small-cell lung cancer. The New England Journal of Medicine. 2015;**372**(21):2018-2028

[48] Gettinger SN et al. Overall survival and long-term safety of Nivolumab (anti-programmed death 1 antibody, BMS-936558, ONO-4538) in patients with previously treated advanced non-small-cell lung cancer. TL - 33. Journal of Clinical Oncology. 2015;**33 VN-r**(18):2004-2012

[49] McDermott DF et al. Survival, durable response, and long-term safety in patients with previously treated advanced renal cell carcinoma receiving Nivolumab. Journal of Clinical Oncology. 2015;**33**(18):2013-2020

[50] Topalian SL et al. Survival, durable tumor remission, and long-term safety in patients with advanced melanoma receiving nivolumab. Journal of Clinical Oncology. Apr. 2014;**32**(10):1020-1030

[51] Farolfi A et al. Ipilimumab in advanced melanoma: Reports of long-lasting responses. Melanoma Research. Jun. 2012;**22**(3):263-270

[52] Keating GM. Nivolumab: A review in advanced squamous non-small cell lung cancer. Drugs. Nov. 2015;**75**(16):1925-1934

[53] Deeks ED. Nivolumab: A review of its use in patients with malignant melanoma. Drugs. Jul. 2014;**74**(11):1233-1239

[54] Larkin J et al. Combined Nivolumab and Ipilimumab or Monotherapy in untreated melanoma. The New England Journal of Medicine. Jul. 2015;**373**(1):23-34

[55] Michot JM et al. Immune-related adverse events with immune checkpoint blockade: A comprehensive review. European Journal of Cancer. Feb. 2016;**54**:139-148

[56] Descotes J. Immunotoxicity of monoclonal antibodies. MAbs. 2009;**1**(2):104-111

[57] Zellner M, Babeluk R, Diestinger M, Pirchegger P, Skeledzic S, Oehler R. Fluorescence-based western blotting for quantitation of protein biomarkers in clinical samples. Electrophoresis. Sep. 2008;**29**(17):3621-3627

[58] Kiyatkin A, Aksamitiene E. Multistrip western blotting to increase quantitative data output. Methods in Molecular Biology. 2009;**536**:149-161

[59] Cho J-YY, Sung H-JJ. Proteomic approaches in lung cancer biomarker development. Expert Review of Proteomics. Feb. 2009;**6**(1):27-42

[60] Tessitore A et al. Serum biomarkers identification by mass spectrometry in high-mortality tumors. International Journal of Proteomics. 2013;**2013**:1-15

[61] Hawkridge AM, Muddiman DC. Mass spectrometry-based biomarker discovery: Toward a global proteome index of individuality. Annual Review of Analytical Chemistry (Palo Alto, California). 2009;**2**:265-277

[62] Ganesan V, Ascherman DP, Minden JS. Immunoproteomics technologies in the discovery of autoantigens in autoimmune diseases. Biomolecular Concepts. May 2016;**7**(2):133-143

[63] Martin K, Ricciardelli C, Hoffmann P, Oehler MK. Exploring the immunoproteome for ovarian cancer biomarker discovery. International Journal of Molecular Sciences. Jan. 2011;**12**(1):410-428

[64] Yuan J et al. Novel technologies and emerging biomarkers for personalized cancer immunotherapy. Journal for ImmunoTherapy of Cancer. 2016;**4**

[65] Broadway N. Recombinant protein expression: Vector-host systems. Materials and Methods. Jun. 2012;**2**:123

[66] Zhu X, Guo A. The critical role of surface chemistry in protein microarrays. Functional Protein Microarrays in Drug Discovery. Boca Raton, FL: CRC Press; 2007. pp. 53-71

[67] Zhu H, Snyder M. Protein chip technology. Current Opinion in Chemical Biology. Feb. 2003;**7**(1):55-63

[68] Patton W. Book reviews: Microarrays and microplates: Applications in biomedical sciences. By S. Ye and I. N. M. Day (editors). Proteomics. Jan. 2003;**3**(1):103-104

[69] Mohamad NRR, Marzuki NHCH, Buang NAA, Huyop F, Wahab RAA. An overview of technologies for immobilization of enzymes and surface analysis techniques for immobilized enzymes. Biotechnology and Biotechnological Equipment. Mar. 2015;**29**(2):205-220

[70] Hu S, Xie Z, Qian J, Blackshaw S, Zhu H. Functional protein microarray technology. Wiley Interdisciplinary Reviews. Systems Biology and Medicine. Sep. 2011;**3**(3):255-268

[71] Tighe PJ, Ryder RR, Todd I, Fairclough LC. ELISA in the multiplex era: Potentials and pitfalls. Proteomics. Clinical Applications. Apr. 2015;**9**(3-4):406-422

[72] Selvarajah S et al. Development and validation of protein microarray technology for simultaneous inflammatory mediator detection in human sera. Mediators of Inflammation. 2014;**2014**

[73] Beeton-Kempen N et al. Development of a novel, quantitative protein microarray platform for the multiplexed serological analysis of autoantibodies to cancer-testis antigens. International Journal of Cancer. Oct. 2014;**135**(8):1842-1851

[74] Nam MJ et al. Molecular profiling of the immune response in colon cancer using protein microarrays: Occurrence of autoantibodies to ubiquitin C-terminal hydrolase L3. Proteomics. Nov. 2003;**3**(11):2108-2115

[75] O'Rourke DJ et al. Autoantibody signatures as biomarkers to distinguish prostate cancer from benign prostatic hyperplasia in patients with increased serum prostate specific antigen. Clinica Chimica Acta. Mar. 2012;**413**(5-6):561-567

[76] Adeola HA, Smith M, Kaestner L, Blackburn JM, Zerbini LF. Novel potential serological prostate cancer biomarkers using CT100+ cancer antigen microarray platform in a multicultural south African cohort. Oncotarget. Mar. 2016;**7**(12):13945-13964

[77] Liew J, Amir A, Chen Y, Fong MYY, Razali R, Lau YLL. Autoantibody profile of patients infected with knowlesi malaria. Clinica Chimica Acta. Aug. 2015;**448**:33-38

[78] Suwarnalata G et al. Augmentation of autoantibodies by helicobacter pylori in Parkinson's disease patients may be linked to greater severity. PLoS One. 2016;**11**(4):1-17

[79] Köhler K, Seitz H. Validation processes of protein biomarkers in serum--a cross platform comparison. Sensors (Basel). 2012;**12**(9):12710-12728

Chapter 11

Development of a Simple Multiplex Electrochemiluminescence (ECL) Assay for Screening Pre-Type 1 Diabetes and Multiple Relevant Autoimmune Diseases

Zhiyuan Zhao, Yong Gu, Jeremy Cheng and Liping Yu

Additional information is available at the end of the chapter

http://dx.doi.org/10.5772/intechopen.75515

Abstract

The presence of islet autoantibodies (iAbs) is currently the most reliable biomarker for type 1 diabetes (T1D). The current "gold" standard radio-binding assays that measure four major iAbs to insulin, IAA, GAD65, IA-2A and ZnT8, are laborious and do not fit for large-scale screenings. Around 40% of patients with T1D develop other autoimmune diseases like celiac disease, autoimmune thyroid disease, and so on. It is highly recommended to screen these closely related autoimmune diseases during T1D screening; however, there is no method available. Recently, on the platform of extensively validated high-sensitive and high-specific electrochemiluminescence (ECL) assay, we developed a multiplex ECL assay to combine up to 10 autoantibody assays into one single well with 5 μl of blood sample. It not only allows us to combine multiple iAbs into one but also makes it possible to simultaneously screen T1D and other multiple autoimmune diseases, which in turn facilitates large-scale screenings in the general population.

Keywords: autoantibody, autoimmune disease, type 1 diabetes, electrochemiluminescence, multuplex assay

1. Introduction

Type 1 diabetes (T1D), the immune-mediated form of diabetes [1], is increasing worldwide, 3–5% annually [2], with rates doubling every 20 years [3, 4], especially in young children.

In the USA, 1.4 million people have T1D and as many have multiple islet autoantibodies (iAbs) or pre-T1D with normal glucose homeostasis. Of the latter, 84% will progress to clinical diabetes in 15 years with a remarkable consistency across populations [5]. Although T1D is a T-lymphocyte-mediated autoimmune disease with specific destruction of pancreatic islet β-cells, autoantibodies directed against proteins in insulin-producing beta cells [1] are the best biomarkers for risk prediction and clinical diagnosis. These iAbs usually appear years before overt clinical disease, and the presence of ≥2 iAbs [antibodies-directed against insulin (IAA), glutamic acid decarboxylase (GADA), islet antigen 2 (IA-2A) or zinc transporter 8 (ZnT8A)] predicts the development of clinical T1D in nearly all affected children [5]. Children at risk for T1D need to be identified prior to the onset of symptoms to: (1) prevent life-threatening diabetic ketoacidosis, (2) identify individuals for current and upcoming trials to prevent T1D and (3) define the onset of islet autoimmunity and its triggers.

Appearance of iAbs is currently the most reliable marker of the autoimmune process leading to T1D, and it determines the disease risk and marks the onset of autoimmune beta cell destruction. The presence of iAbs, their number [6–8] and titer [9–11], has being used extensively to stage diabetes risk and as inclusion criteria into T1D prevention trials [12]. Immunoassays to detect iAbs can be classified into four generations. The first generation is the indirect immunofluorescence on cryostat sections of the pancreas for islet cell antibodies (ICA) [13, 14] present in patients' sera to a variety of autoantigens in islet β-cells. This assay requires the pancreas tissue to conduct the measurement and is very limited in the regular screening. The second generation of iAbs immunoassays is a well-established radio-binding assay (RBA) which is based on various biochemically defined autoantigens and plays a major role as the current gold standard assay for all four major islet autoantibodies IAA, GADA, IA-2A and ZnT8A and ELISAs. Traditional ELISA has been proved not to work well for any iAbs with less sensitivity and less specific in multiple workshops of Islet Autoantibody Standardization Program (IASP, previously DASP). However, a modified bridging ELISA with semifluid-phase interaction between the antibody and antigen has achieved sensitivity and specificity equivalent to the RBA for the measurement of GADA, IA-2A and ZnT8A [15–19]. The third generation is a recently developed and extensively validated nonradioactive iAb assay using electrochemiluminescence (ECL) detection with a higher sensitivity and higher disease specificity compared to the RBAs [20–25]. The ECL assay has been demonstrated to be more sensitive and is able to identify the first iAb of "seroconversion" earlier than RBA by years in young children followed from the birth on pre-T1D who were followed to clinical diabetes. More remarkably, ECL assay is able to discriminate high-affinity, high-risk autoantibodies from those "low risk," low-affinity signals generated by RBA in subjects with single iAb who are less likely to progress to T1D. The fourth generation of autoantibody immunoassays is to develop a simple multiplexed assay to fit for the needs of ongoing and future clinical trials to simultaneously screen multiple iAbs and other autoantibodies in one single well, which will facilitate high-throughput autoantibody screening simultaneously for T1D and other multiple relevant autoimmune diseases in large scale of populations. ECL assay has been illustrated as an excellent platform for a simple multiplex assay with a superior advantage of high sensitivity and disease specificity. In this chapter, we mainly focus on the discussion of: (1) two currently most popular assays for iAbs, a gold standard RBA and a modified bridging ELISA; (2) ECL assay and its comparison with RBA and (3) development of a simple multiplex ECL assay with all advantages considered.

2. Radio-binding assay (RBA) and enzyme-linked immunosorbent assay (ELISA)

At present, four major biochemically defined β-cell autoantigens were well characterized including IAA [26], GAD65 [27], IA-2 [28] and ZnT8 [29]. Through laboratory proficiency programs [30, 31] and harmonization efforts [32], RBA, a fluid-phase assay using radiolabeled antigens and precipitating antibody-antigen complex by Protein A/G Sepharose, has been well established as a current "gold" standard assay for autoantibodies to all four major antigens [29, 32, 33].

In RBA, recombinant human insulin is labeled with I-125, while GAD, IA-2 and ZnT8 antigens are expressed from their corresponding recombinant human cDNA and labeled with 35S-methionine by coupled in vitro transcription/translation. To assess general implementation of assay methods and to standardize the iAb assays, the Center for Disease Control and Prevention (CDC) and Immunology and Diabetes Society (IDS) started organizing the Diabetes Autoantibody Standardization Program (DASP) workshop in the year of 2000 [34]. Forty-six laboratories in 13 countries participated in the program. The first proficiency evaluation of DASP showed a high concordance in measurement of GADA ($r = 0.96$; $p < 0.0001$) and IA-2A ($r = 0.89$; $p < 0.0001$) using the new WHO international reference reagent. In contrast, the workshop demonstrated wide variation among IAA assays, with poor overall performance and low sensitivity. IAA assays were improved after the first proficiency evaluation and the median laboratory assigned sensitivity was 26, 36 and 45% in 2002, 2003 and 2005, respectively ($p < 0.0001$). However, the IAA assay has proven the most difficult to standardize with relatively wide discrepancies between laboratories in the IASP workshop and has not yet achieved a satisfactory level of sensitivity and specificity. There was still remarkable variation between laboratories and the ranking of IAA levels in patient serum samples was concordant to AUC ($p < 0.001$), and the AUC ranged from 0.36 to 0.91 [30]. To facilitate comparison of quantitative islet autoantibody results between studies, the National Institute of Diabetes and Digestive and Kidney Diseases (NIDDK) set up an Islet Autoantibody Harmonization Committee in 2007 to align measurement and reporting of iAbs in all NIDDK-sponsored studies and several different central laboratories are used [32]. With a few years of combined efforts, both GADA and IA-2A assays were successfully harmonized with great concordance as positive or negative between participating laboratories. The IA-2A assay, using a common threshold of 5 DK units/ml, achieved 64% sensitivity with specificity greater than 99% in all laboratories. For GADA, using thresholds equivalent to the 97th percentile of 974 control samples in each laboratory, 1051 (97.9%) of 1074 samples were concordant. ZnT8 is a most recently identified new islet β-cell autoantigen, and ZnT8A assay has been well established through IASP workshop. In combination of current four iAb assays by the standard RBA, the overall sensitivity is able to cover around 95% in newly diagnosed patients with T1D [29]. To lead to more reproducible identification of individuals at risk of type 1 diabetes and improve monitoring in long-term prospective studies, some recommendations by the Islet Autoantibody Harmonization Committee have been applied to current national and international clinical trials for T1D: (1) confirmation of positive results in a second laboratory is likely to be valuable to identify discrepancies; (2) laboratories should use common calibrators against reference standards; (3) the methods used in multiple centers should be compared and harmonized to eliminate potential factors that will contribute to discrepancies; (4) a common set of samples which can provide knowledge of concordance, sensitivity and specificity including a large number of samples from healthy controls, and patients should be identified to establish working thresholds of positivity that are similar between the participating laboratories.

T1D is now able to be predicted by measuring iAbs present in the peripheral blood, and these iAbs have been used to determine disease risk and onset of autoimmune beta cell destruction. Almost all children with two or more of these iAbs will progress to clinical diabetes with a remarkable consistency across populations, while progression to diabetes in children persistently positive for a single iAb is only 15% in 15 years [30], as most of these children have a low-affinity iAb not associated with disease [35–37].

In summary, the current method most commonly used for screening iAbs is the "gold" standard RBA, a fluid-phase assay using radiolabeled antigens and immunoprecipitation, to quantify four major iAbs named IAA, GADA, IA-2A and ZNT8A. These four RBAs are currently able to cover 95% of sensitivity in newly diagnosed patients with T1D. Through the efforts of iAb proficiency programs and harmonization consortia, current standard RBA for iAbs have been greatly improved, but there are still work to be done, especially (1) IAA is not achieved its sensitivity and specificity and (2) there is a low risk prediction in subjects with single iAb positivity.

A direct enzyme-linked immunosorbent assay (ELISA) format (binding of antigen to plate and detection of bound autoantibody with labeled anti-antibodies) has proven difficult to develop. To date, only one ELISA-based ElisaRSR™ for GADA, IA-2A and ZnT8A, distributed by Kronus that utilizes capture of solution-phase antigen by one chain of immunoglobulin (Ig) while being bound by its other chain to plate-bound antigen has demonstrated sensitivity and specificity similar to the fluid-phase RBA (www.rsrltd.com). But there is no any ELISA-based assay that works well for IAA measurement according to IASP workshop [30]. ELISA assays were found only to detect insulin antibodies induced by exogenous insulin injection [38], but not natural insulin autoantibodies. Our group reported a high sensitive ELISA-based competition Europium IAA assay in 2009 [39], and it worked very well for mouse IAA assay, but unfortunately it did not work at all for human samples, although RBA-IAA assay works equally well for both human and mouse samples [33].

3. Electrochemiluminescence (ECL) assays

While the current standard RBA for iAbs has been greatly improved through the laboratory proficiency programs and harmonization efforts, there are still works in progress. The IAA assay, especially, has not yet achieved a satisfactory level of sensitivity and specificity. Importantly, IAA has a high prevalence among young children [36] and is usually the first iAb to appear in young children [37]. The ability of prospective clinical studies, for example, The Environmental Determinants of Diabetes in the Young (TEDDY), which aims to identify triggers of islet autoimmunity, depends on accurate detection of the timing of appearance of the first iAb to mark the very beginning of islet autoimmunity. We have recently developed and extensively validated a new generation of nonradioactive iAb assay using ECL detection, as we described in the previous section, with an excellent sensitivity and specificity [20–25] for both IAA and GADA. The assay is based on the principle that interaction of autoantibodies with antigen molecules is in liquid phase, and the detection signals are directly from the labeled antigen molecules bound to specific autoantibodies without applying the labeled second antibody (labeled anti-human IgG antibody usually used in conventional ELISA) for detection, which usually causes a very high background in autoantibody assays with human samples. As illustrated for ECL assay protocol in **Figure 1**, autoantibodies in serum help bridge the Sulfo-tagged antigen molecule to the biotinylated antigen molecule, which will be captured on the solid phase of the streptavidin-coated plate. Detection of plate-captured Sulfo-tagged antigen is accomplished with electrochemiluminescence. The fact that the ECL assay is able to capture all immunoglobulin subgroups no matter IgG, IgM, IgA or IgE allows this assay a higher sensitivity than current standard RBA based on IgG detection. With the new ECL assays, we have analyzed thousands of participants in Diabetes Autoimmunity Study in the Young (DAISY) [21], TrialNet Pathway to Prevention subjects [23] and very recently TEDDY subjects (unpublished data). Compared with gold standard RBA, the ECL assays, especially ECL-IAA assays, were demonstrated more sensitive. In DAISY longitudinally follow-up study, we analyzed 427 sequential samples from 63 pre-T1D who were closely followed to clinical T1D. Nearly all of these children (62/63) were detected ECL-IAA years before disease onset, including 10 children who were completely IAA negative by RBA-IAA during the follow-up. Remarkably, 25% of these early longitudinally followed samples during

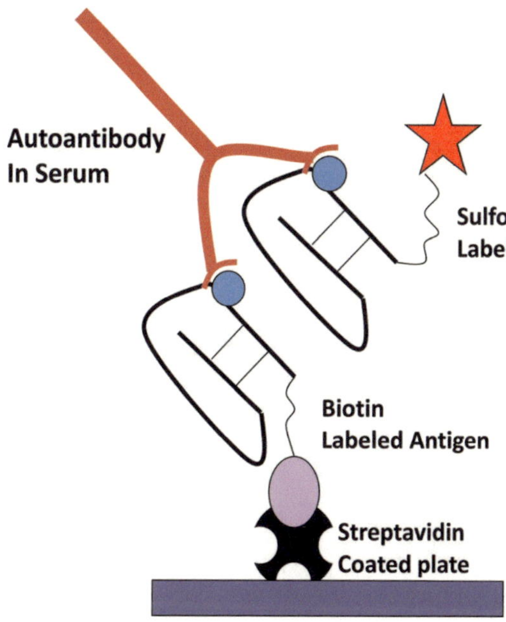

Figure 1. Illustration of the bivalent plate capture ECL assay. The antibody in serum will link the Sulfo-tagged antigen to the biotinylated antigen, which will be captured on the solid phase of the streptavidin-coated plate. Detection of plate-captured Sulfo-tagged antigen is accomplished with electrochemiluminescence.

pre-diabetes stage which were positive for ECL-IAA were negative for RBA-IAA (**Figure 2**). ECL-IAA were found to antedate the onset of islet autoimmunity in these children by a mean of 2.3 years (range: 0.3–7.2 years) [21]. The earlier identification of IAA among young children was validated from a later TEDDY study cohort (unpublished data). Results from these studies indicate that this novel ECL-IAA assay is not only more sensitive but also defines the timing of the initial autoantibody appearance earlier than the previously used RBA-IAA. This earlier detection and accuracy in timing of onset of islet autoimmunity in young children followed from the birth is important to find potential environmental causes of diabetes and our understanding of the etiology of T1D as the ability to identify triggers of islet autoimmunity, for example, TEDDY study depends on the sensitivity and validity of iAb assays used to pinpoint the "seroconversion" to islet autoimmunity.

Remarkably, both ECL-IAA and ECL-GADA assays were selectively detecting the positivity from the high-risk subjects who were followed to progression of clinical T1D or the subjects who were multiple iAbs positive. In the study of DAISY children [20, 22], we analyzed all pre-T1D children who were followed to clinical diabetes and all non-diabetic children who were persistently iAbs positive, either multiple iAbs or single iAb, and compared them with RBA. Almost all samples positive by RBA (IAA or GADA) were ECL assay positive in children on pre-T1D or children with presence of multiple iAbs. In contrast, only around 25% of non-diabetic children with either single IAA or single GADA positive by RBA were ECL positive. **Figure 3** shows positivity of IAA among some children in the DAISY study as an example, persistently expressing IAA with other iAbs (multiple iAbs) or as a single iAb. Panel A: ECL-IAA

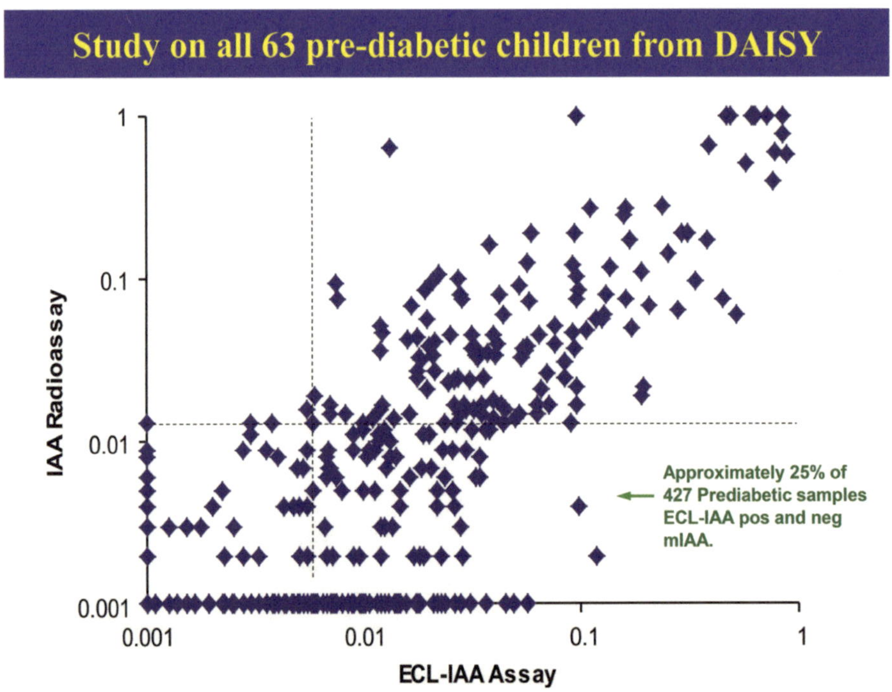

Figure 2. IAA identification in pre-diabetic children by ECL-IAA. The x-axis represents results of ECL-IAA assay and the y-axis represents results of mIAA RIA assay. About 25% of pre-diabetic samples were positive for ECL-IAA but negative for mIAA RIA assay.

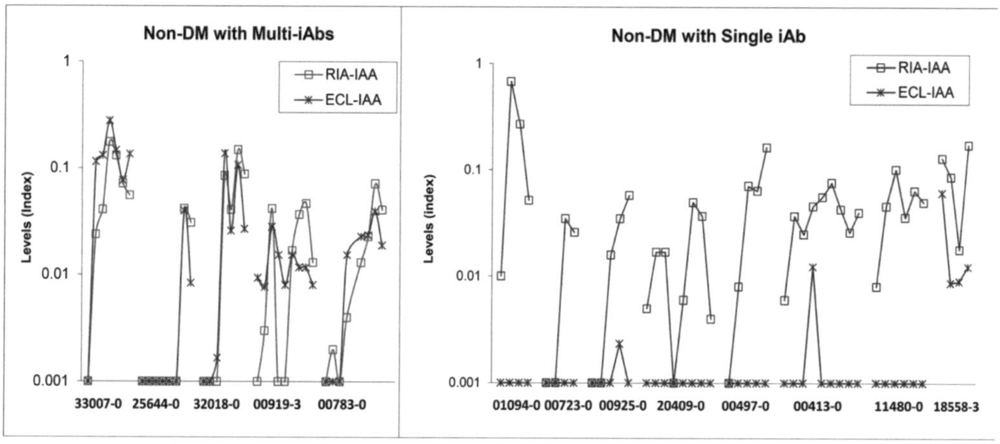

Panel A Panel B

Figure 3. Sera from children in the DAISY study persistently expressing IAA as a single or with multiple iAbs were analyzed with the ECL-IAA assay. Panel A: ECL-IAA was well correlated with RBA-IAA for all 5 subjects (multiple follow-up positive for both assays) who were multiple iAbs positive. Panel B: 7/8 subjects with single iAb (IAA only) were consistently ECL-IAA negative.

was well correlated with RBA-IAA for all five subjects (multiple follow-up positive for both assays), who were multiple iAbs positive. Panel B: 7/8 subjects with single iAb (IAA only) were consistently ECL-IAA negative. The antibody affinity study was performed to compare these IAA or GADA detected by RBA, but differentiated by ECL assay as positive or negative. The results of affinity analysis discovered that IAA or GADA detected by RBA, but negative with ECL assay, in children who were absent of other iAbs had low affinity, while IAA or GADA positive by both RBA and ECL assays had high affinity. **Figure 4** illustrates the IAA (panel A) or GADA (panel B) competition assays with unlabeled proinsulin or GAD65 protein. The IAA or GADA not detected by the ECL assay required a 10- to 100-fold higher concentration of unlabeled insulin/proinsulin or GAD65 protein for 50% inhibition of binding of IAA or GADA to labeled insulin or GAD65 protein. These results demonstrated that both ECL-IAA and ECL-GADA were able to discriminate high-affinity, high-risk iAbs from those "low risk," low-affinity signals generated by RBA in subjects who are less likely to progress to T1D. In our later validation study with a large TrialNet cohort of Pathway to Prevention, identical results were obtained [23] by characteristics of disease specificity with both ECL-IAA and ECL-GADA. The study analyzed 3500 subjects in blind with 571 multiple iAbs, 1727 single iAb and 384 pre-T1D who were followed to clinical T1D later in the study. The ECL assay and RBA were found congruent in pre-diabetics and in the subjects with multiple autoantibodies, but only 24% of single RBA-IAA ($p < 0.0001$) and 46% of single RBA-GADA ($p < 0.0001$) were confirmed by the ECL-IAA and ECL-GADA assays, respectively. With the prospective following up for the subjects with single IAA or GADA, 51% of RBA-IAA and 63% of RBA-GADA subjects not confirmed by ECL were found lost their iAbs and became iAb negative after a mean follow-up time of 2.4 years, behaving as "transient" iAb positivity. Only a few subjects converted to multiple iAbs or progressed to clinical diabetes. In contrast, only small percentages of RBA-IAA and RBA-GADA confirmed by ECL assays became negative ($p < 0.0001$ for both IAA and GADA) during the follow-up as significant number of subjects progressed to clinical diabetes or multiple iAbs. In the study, 2944 subjects were studied with their very first initial screening samples

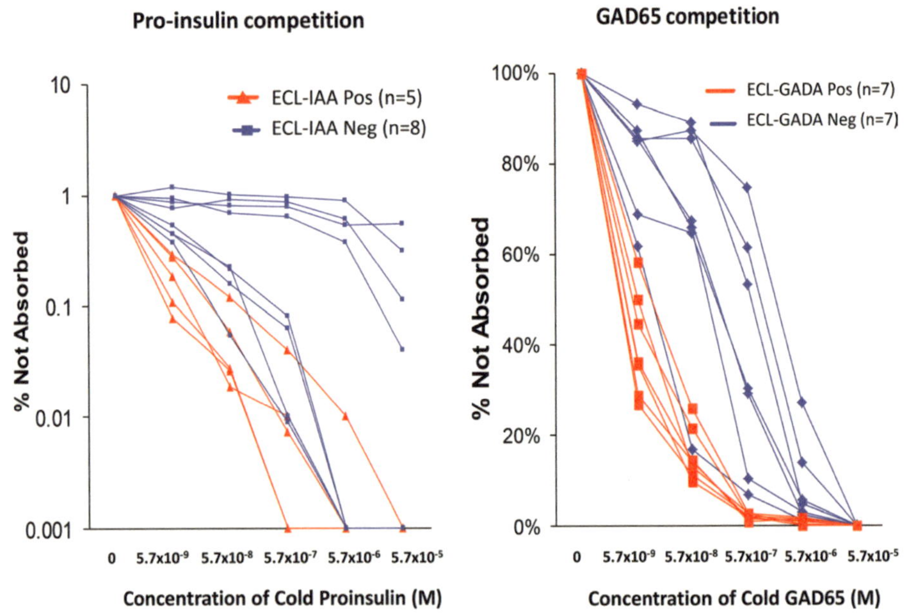

Figure 4. Illustration of the IAA (Panel A) or GADA (Panel B) competition assays with unlabeled proinsulin or GAD65 protein. IAA /GADA negative by ECL-IAA / ECL-GADA assay (blue line), compared with IAA /GADA positive by ECL-GADA/ECL-IAA assay (red line), and required higher concentrations of unlabeled insulin/proinsulin or GAD65 protein for 50% maximal inhibition, which is consistent with low affinity.

and prospectively followed to clinical T1D during the study period. The positive and negative predictive values of RBA and ECL assays, in terms of progression to T1D, were analyzed and compared, and the data are illustrated in **Figure 5**. The positive predictive values for ECL-IAA and ECL-GADA were 32 and 24%, significantly higher than those RBA-IAA and RBA-GADA (21 and 16%, respectively; both $p < 0.0001$) (panel A). Similarly, the negative predictive values for ECL-IAA and ECL-GADA were 94 and 96%, significantly higher than those for RBA-IAA and RBA-GADA (92%; $p < 0.05$ and 94%; $p = 0.007$, respectively) (panel B). Compared with HLA analysis, the highest risk genotype for T1D, HLA-DR3/4, DQB1*0302 was significantly higher in subjects with IAA or GADA confirmed by ECL than those not confirmed by ECL assays ($p < 0.0017$ and $p < 0.0001$, respectively). The frequency of this high-risk HLA genotype in subjects with either single IAA or GADA not confirmed by ECL assays was found identical to subjects with negative results for all iAbs, a very low-risk population who are very unlikely to progress to T1D.

Autoantibody affinity in sequential follow-up samples from their initial positive screening to their later follow-up with a mean follow-up of 5.3 years were investigated [25] in a subset of subjects in TrialNet Pathway to Prevention study who were persistent single RBA-IAA or single RBA-GADA positive confirmed or not confirmed by ECL assays. Among either single IAA or single GADA subjects, all subjects who were confirmed by ECL assays were found to have high affinity autoantibodies at their very first initial positive visit. Affinity results stayed consistent over time. Similarly, those who were negative for ECL assays showed lower affinity at initial visit and affinity stayed low over time. No converting events from low to high or high

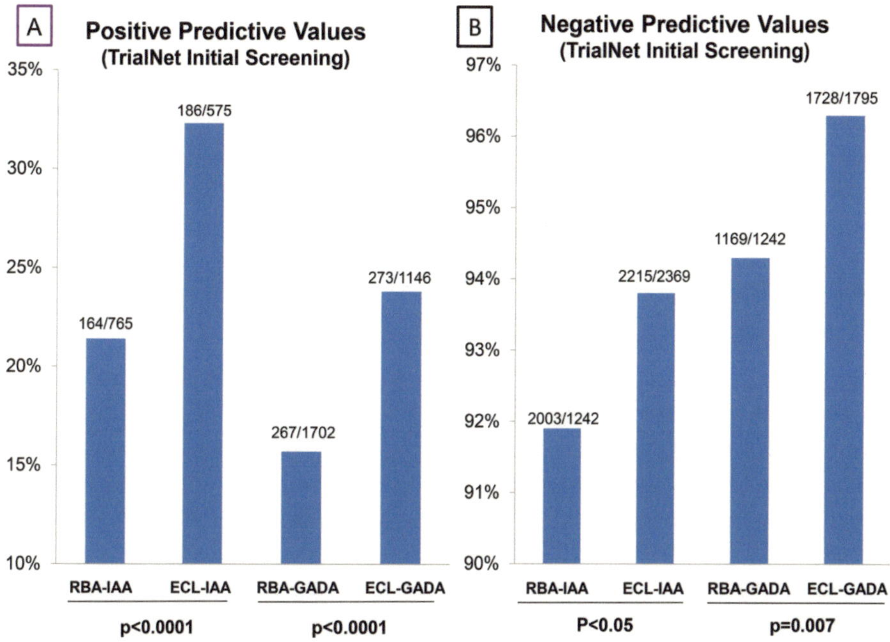

Figure 5. Predictive values of IAA and GADA assays in the TrialNet Initial Screening study. A: Positive predictive values of RIA-IAA and ECL-IAA assays, RIA-GADA and ECL-GADA assays. B: Negative predictive values of RIA-IAA and ECL-IAA assays, RIA-GADA and ECL-GADA assays. Positive and negative predictive values of ECL-IAA and ECL-GADA were significantly higher than those of RIA-IAA and RIA-GADA assays, respectively.

to low affinity were seen over time. There were 14 subjects in the group who progressed to clinical T1D during the study period. All except one were ECL-positive and had a high affinity for IAA or GADA. These results implicate that a more disease-specific iAb measurement like ECL assay can identify high affinity iAbs with high disease risk on the early stage of initial screening. It is generally assumed that the very low risk of those with only a single iAb, either single IAA or single GADA, spreading of autoimmunity to other autoantigens is needed to increase risk or marks a stage closer to overt diabetes, and multiple studies of both relatives of T1D patients and general populations have documented that expression of multiple iAbs are associated with extreme risk of progression to T1D. The pattern of expression of iAbs detected by ECL assays predicts both epitope spreading and diabetes risk. Differences in iAbs reactivity can be assessed prior to epitope spreading consistent with early determination of both

	RBA positive, GADA only			RBA positive, IAA only		
	ECL+ (n = 107)	ECL− (n = 78)	p-value	ECL+ (n = 24)	ECL− (n = 63)	p-value
PS6M (mg/dl)	22 ± 90	−19 ± 71	0.001	36 ± 75	−9 ± 70	0.009
Progressed to T1D	14.0% (n = 15)	1.3% (n = 1)	0.002	16.7% (n = 4)	0% (n = 0)	0.005

PS6M is a 6-month progression scale based on worsening of the 30–120-min OGTT glucose.

Table 1. ECL iAb identify progressors to T1D among children and adults with single iAb by RBA.

epitope spreading and diabetes risk. This is of particular value in children and young adults who are positive for a single iAb, as demonstrated by TrialNet Pathway to Prevention (**Table 1**, J Sosenko, manuscript submitted). Among TrialNet participants who were positive for a single iAb by RBA, 52% (141/272) were not confirmed by ECL. These ECL-negative subjects showed no worsening of glycemia and little progression to T1D during a median follow-up of 4.7 years. In contrast, OGTT glycemia worsened significantly in the ECL-positive single iAb participants, comparably with the worsening in 90 multiple iAb + subjects (PS6M 23 ± 96 mg/dl); the latter group had a high risk for progression to T1D (30%). The ECL assay can substantially refine the selection of single iAb positive individuals at high risk, who possibly could be recruited for participation in T1D prevention trials.

Presently, clinical prevention trials in T1D TrialNet study are only selecting relatives of patients with T1D who have multiple iAbs. It is generally agreed that some clinical intervening on early stages of islet autoimmune processes could result in a better outcome as some evidence in animal model for prevention [40], but the clinical trial studies using subjects with single iAb, either single IAA or GADA, are not available since the risk is too low. However, the subjects with single iAb (IAA or GADA) detected by more disease-specific assays like ECL assay with the nature of ability to detect high affinity antibodies may qualify for enrollment into prevention trials as their risk for diabetes is much higher and those with low affinity, low-risk signals generated by RBA will be removed [20, 22, 23, 25]. On the other hand, subjects found to be negative for ECL assays may benefit from less intensive monitoring in these longitudinal prospective studies [41] to save the efforts and costs of these studies.

In summary, islet autoimmunity of T1D can be identified at the very beginning of the disease process by measurements of iAbs. Two major iAbs, IAA and GADA, usually appear earlier than other iAbs and are often detected in isolation as single iAb in the screening of relatives and general population. Most of these single iAbs detected by current gold standard RBA are at low risk, low affinity and non-disease relevant as "biologically" false positives while part of these single iAbs does represent the early stage of islet autoimmunity in T1D progression. With more disease-specific assays like an ECL assay method, high-risk and disease-relevant iAbs are able to be identified at the very beginning of the disease process in subjects with single iAb before the development of multiple iAbs closer to overt clinical diabetes, which will be greatly appreciated for clearing the current confusions of single iAb positivity and aid the T1D clinical trials for both identifying environmental triggers of islet autoimmunity and intervening with islet autoimmune process on very beginning stage to prevent the disease. The ECL assay was demonstrated its superiority to RBA in sensitivity and especially ECL-IAA was able to antedated the onset of islet autoimmunity by years than RBA, which will be very important to accurately pinpoint the very beginning of islet autoimmunity for identifying the environmental triggers to cause the T1D.

4. Development of a multiplex assay for large-scale screening

At present, many large-scale national and international clinical trials for T1D are in progress, and multiple candidate interventions are being proposed to abrogate or slow progression of T1D among iAb positive subjects. A wider screening of iAbs in the general population, especially in young children, is perspectively in progress or in planning. Currently, four biochemically defined iAbs including IAA, GADA, IA-2A and ZnT8A are equally important in prediction and evaluation of risk of progression to T1D in both relatives of patients with T1D and general population. The screening methods using current standard RBA with single iAb measurement are laborious and inefficient for such a large scale of screening. While significant progress has been made in standardization of iAb assays and high-throughput technologies, the cost and logistic complexity of currently used methods preclude their widespread use in population-based screening. The determination of initial iAb positivity is very important, which may represent the initiation of islet autoimmunity. However, the results of iAb measurement at this early stage in subjects with a single iAb are not reliable with current standard RBA since the majority of these single iAb subjects identified by RBA have low affinity antibodies, most of them transient, and therefore biologically appear to be "false positives" with respect to T1D development as we discussed earlier. Poor assay specificity is likely to be more problematic for screening process in general population with lower frequency of risk for T1D than high risk relative cohort as in TrialNet Pathway to Prevention we studied. A high-throughput assay technology with improved disease specificity will be important and necessary.

One in four children at risk for T1D develops islet, celiac, thyroid or rheumatoid autoimmunity in the DAISY study. Interestingly, there is little overlap of these phenotypes in an individual child, but this overlap increases with age. The incidence of autoantibodies to thyroid peroxidase (TPOA) surges after the age of 12. Importantly, up to 40% of patients with T1D have an additional autoimmune condition [42–44]. It is important and urgent to screen biomarkers of other autoimmune diseases when screening diabetes, simultaneously. Unfortunately, there is no easy and inexpensive tool to screen for these conditions. With a big effort, all DAISY and TEDDY study participants are screened for autoantibodies to tissue transglutaminase (TGA) for celiac disease autoimmunity. Persistent TGA positivity and celiac disease are secondary endpoints in both studies [45, 46]. DAISY data suggest that, by age 18, at least 7% of the general population persistently express one or more of the nine autoantibodies: IAA, GADA, IA-2A, ZnT8A, TPOA, TGA and three other autoantibodies for rheumatoid arthritis, Addison's disease and autoimmune gastritis. If confirmed, this would argue for a universal screening. We have carried out a pilot of such screening for iAbs and TGA, in children of 2–6 years old attending general pediatric care offices in Denver [47]. Participating parents and providers ranked the combined screening for iAbs and TGA as more valuable than screening for iAbs alone.

To fit the purpose of large-scale screening in national clinical trials and the general population, people are starting to seek a possible method of a multiplexed assay combining multiple autoantibody assays together in one single well. Recently, a few studies of multiplex antibody assays were reported with different technologies [48–51], but none of these assay platforms has neither compared with currently used "gold" standard RBA for its sensitivity and specificity in T1D study, especially in subjects with risk to T1D, nor validated in an international Islet Autoantibody Standardization Program (IASP) workshop or in a large cohort of clinical trial. From previous multiple studies, none of the conventional ELISA methods worked well for any iAb measurements, especially for IAA according to multiple IASP workshop [30]. Interaction of iAbs with their corresponding antigen proteins in liquid phase will still be necessary in a multiplex assay setting to achieve a proper sensitivity and specificity and it is a particularly essential condition for IAA assay. The capacity of specific autoantibody-antigen binding might be a new consideration with our recent experiences in a multiplex assay setting, which has never been an issue in any single antibody assay format. Multiple autoantibody-antigen interactions share the space within one single well in a multiplex assay setting, and each of these interactions might need enough number of their own specific antibodies binding to their corresponding antigen proteins to generate a signal strong enough to be detected, which is particularly important when these autoantibodies are at low levels.

Very recently, a modified ELISA-based ElisaRSR™ 3-Screen ICA™ is now available for research from the RSR Limited (3-Screen ICA™ ELISA; www.rsrltd.com). It is a combination assay for measuring GADA, IA-2A and ZnT8A. Its single assay platform was validated at multiple IASP workshops for its sensitivity and specificity. The 3 Screen ELISA assay measures three autoantibodies either in three separate wells consuming large volume of serum or in one single well with three assays mixed not able to distinguish which of the three beta cell autoantibodies are present. The biggest disadvantage of the 3 Screen ELISA is its inability to include IAA measurement in the assay. IAA has a very high rate of positivity in young children and is considered as the first iAb on early stages of islet autoimmunity as we discussed earlier. Compared with current single iAb RBA or original single ELISA-based ElisaRSR™ assays, the 3 Screen ELISA assay definitely has its advantage of higher efficiency [52], but screening with its own without including IAA measurement will be a big defect and will not be the best way to persume.

With the platform of our newly established ECL assay technology, we recently published our study of a multiplex assay to accurately measure four autoantibodies in one single well [53] with MesoScale Discovery (MSD) QuickPlex 4-Spot plate as illustrated in

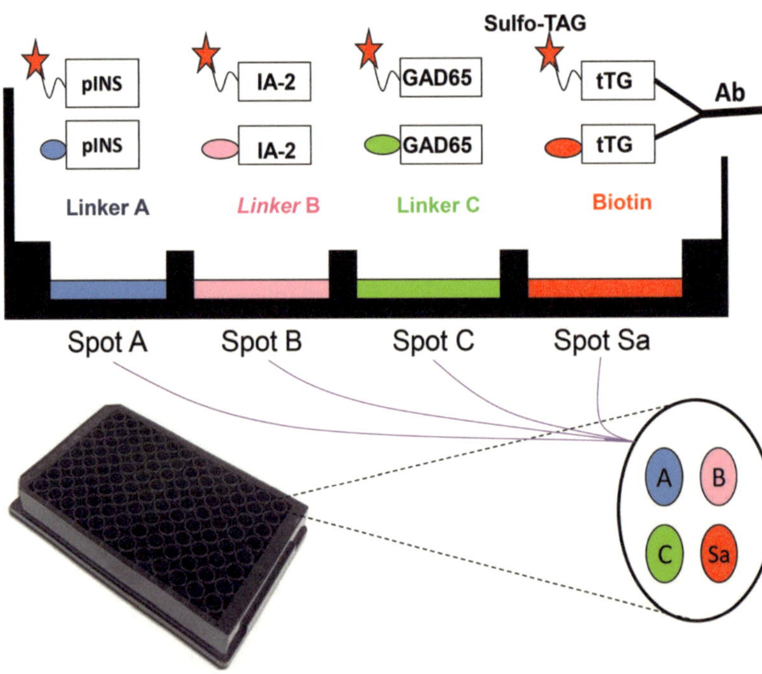

Figure 6. Illustration of ECL 4-spot assay. The 4-spot assay is based on the same mechanism of single ECL assay. Each biotinylated antigen will be linked by its corresponding linker which will be captured on the solid phase of the pre-coated plate. Detection of plate-captured Sulfo-tagged antigen is also accomplished with electrochemiluminescence. 4-spot assay is able to accommodate up to 4 autoantibody assays in one well.

Figure 6. The 4-plex assay was based on the same mechanism of our single ECL assay, but linker system was introduced. Four interactions of antibody-antigen are, respectively, restrained on each of four specific linker spots within the same well, and the camera is able to catch the signals from four different sources of spots, respectively. With the limitation of four spots able to accommodate maximum four autoantibody assays in one well, we selected, on purposely, IAA, GADA, IA-2A and TGA. We included TGA instead of ZnT8A because (1) ZnT8A is almost always present with other iAbs and ZnT8A alone is only 1% in subject followed to T1D (8). In two large national clinical trials of TrialNet and TEDDY, ZnT8A is not included in intial screening, and the ZnT8A assay is only performed if any of other three iAbs is positive. (2) We want to screen both T1D and celiac disease as we rationaled earlier. The 4-plex assay retained 100% sensitivity and 100% specificity for all four autoantibodies in terms of positivity identified in patients versus normal controls compared to the corresponding standard RBA and our single ECL assays. In early 2015, MSD company released the new U-Plex™ Development Packs system for creating custom multiplex panels of analytes to replace the QuickPlex 4-Spot system. With a similar principle of multiplex assay mechanism of QuickPlex 4-Spot system, this new system expanded multiplexing up to 10, combining 10 different autoantibody assays in one single well with the same amount of 6 μl serum sample used for a single ECL assay. The UPlex plate assay system is illustrated in **Figure 7** as we currently used it as an UPlex 8-plex assay. With this new system, we have successfully combined eight autoantibody assays within one single well including all four iAbs and four other

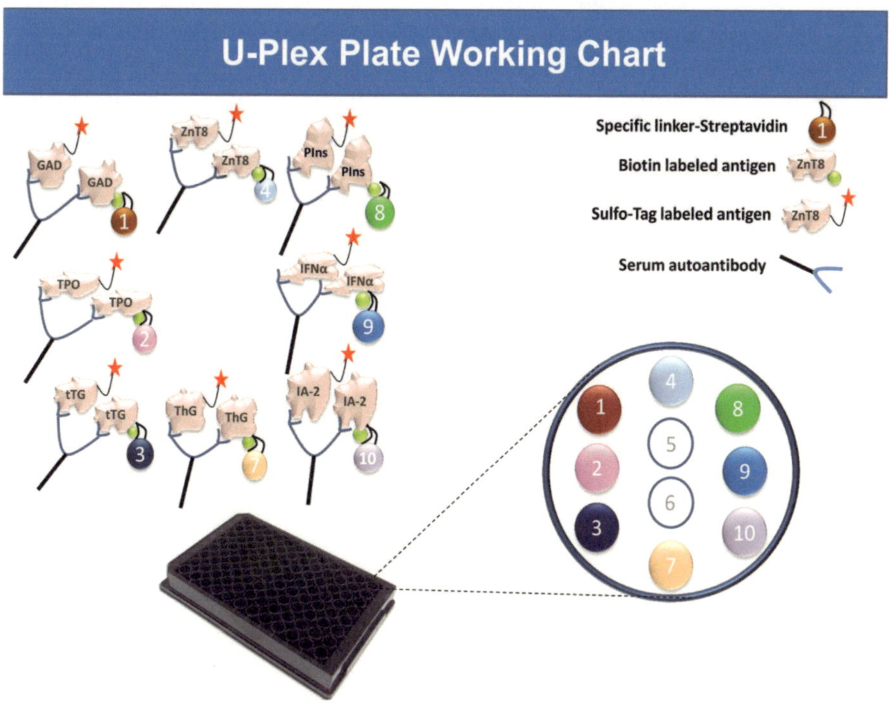

Figure 7. Illustration of UPlex 8-plex plate working chart. 8-plex assay is working on the same mechanism of 4-spot assay. Uplex can combine up to 10 antibody assays in one well.

autoantibody assays, TGA for celiac disease, TPOA and autoantibodies to thyroid globulin (ThGA) for autoimmune thyroiditis, autoantibodies to interferon alpha (IFNaA) for autoimmune polyglandular syndrom-1 (APS-1). With 100th percentile of specificity in 118 healthy normal controls, the 8-plex assay was able to retain 100% sensitivity for all autoantibodies, and the levels of autoantibodies in 8-plex assay were well correlated with their corresponding single RBA or ELISA (for IFNaA) in 168 T1D patients. The further work of assay optimization needs to be done to minimize the interferences of cross-talking between spots, especially an extreme high signal on one spot overspilled to a neighboring spot when it should be negative. The UPlex system made it possible to customize a multiplexed assay according to the needs for screening. It is capable to screen children simultaneously for T1D and other multiple autoimmune diseases often happening in childhood. It is also capable to screen adults simultaneously for T1D and other multiple autoimmune diseases usually seen in adulthood. Such a multiplex ECL assay technology will retain high assay sensitivity and disease specificity as we discussed earlier and provide a great tool for a large scale of screening in the general population with high efficiency and low cost using only a tiny amount of blood sample. We expect these multiplex assays with new technologies, be available in clinic and easily applied for population screening in the near future.

In conclusion, T1D is now predictable by measuring major iAbs. The ECL assay for iAbs is superior to the current gold standard RBA and other methods in terms of assay sensitivity and specificity for disease risk prediction. With a rapid increasing rate of disease, large scales of population screenings are becoming important for the public health. Large percent of patients with T1D develop other autoimmune diseases, and it has been recommended to screen other relevant automimmune diseases when screening diabetes autoimmunity simultaneously. With the advantages of the ECL assay in its nature of high assay sensitivity and high disease specificity, a simple multiplex assay built on the platform of ECL technology will provide an excellent tool to not only screen multiple iAbs in one single well, but also screen multiple autoimmune diseases simultaneously in large scale of populations efficiently and economically.

Acknowledgements

This study is supported by JDRF grants 2-SRA-2015-2051-Q-R and 2-SRA-2018-533-S-B; NIH grant DK32083; Diabetes Autoimmunity Study in the Young Grant DK32493.

Author details

Zhiyuan Zhao, Yong Gu, Jeremy Cheng and Liping Yu*

*Address all correspondence to: Liping.yu@ucdenver.edu

Barbara Davis Center for Childhood Diabetes, University of Colorado School of Medicine, Aurora, CO, USA

References

[1] Atkinson MA, Eisenbarth GS, Michels AW. Type 1 diabetes. Lancet. 2014;**383**(9911):69-82

[2] Secular trends in incidence of childhood IDDM in 10 countries. Diabetes Epidemiology Research International Group. Diabetes. 1990;**39**(7):858-864

[3] Harjutsalo V, Sjoberg L, Tuomilehto J. Time trends in the incidence of type 1 diabetes in Finnish children: A cohort study. Lancet. 2008;**371**(9626):1777-1782

[4] Vehik K et al. Increasing incidence of type 1 diabetes in 0- to 17-year-old Colorado youth. Diabetes Care. 2007;**30**(3):503-509

[5] Ziegler AG et al. Seroconversion to multiple islet autoantibodies and risk of progression to diabetes in children. JAMA. 2013;**309**(23):2473-2479

[6] Orban T et al. Pancreatic islet autoantibodies as predictors of type 1 diabetes in the Diabetes Prevention Trial-Type 1. Diabetes Care. 2009;**32**(12):2269-2274

[7] Bingley PJ. Clinical applications of diabetes antibody testing. Journal of Clinical Endo crinology and Metabolism. 2010;**95**(1):25-33

[8] Yu L et al. Zinc transporter-8 autoantibodies improve prediction of type 1 diabetes in relatives positive for the standard biochemical autoantibodies. Diabetes Care. 2012;**35**(6): 1213-1218

[9] Steck AK et al. Age of islet autoantibody appearance and mean levels of insulin, but not GAD or IA-2 autoantibodies, predict age of diagnosis of type 1 diabetes: Diabetes autoimmunity study in the young. Diabetes Care. 2011;**34**(6):1397-1399

[10] Sosenko JM et al. A longitudinal study of GAD65 and ICA512 autoantibodies during the progression to type 1 diabetes in Diabetes Prevention Trial-Type 1 (DPT-1) participants. Diabetes Care. 2011;**34**(11):2435-2437

[11] Sosenko JM et al. The prediction of type 1 diabetes by multiple autoantibody levels and their incorporation into an autoantibody risk score in relatives of type 1 diabetic patients. Diabetes Care. 2013;**36**(9):2615-2620

[12] Vehik K et al. Islet autoantibody seroconversion in the DPT-1 study: Justification for repeat screening throughout childhood. Diabetes Care. 2011;**34**(2):358-362

[13] Pollard DR et al. An immunofluorescence study of anti-pancreatic islet cell antibodies in the spontaneously diabetic BB Wistar rat. Diabetologia. 1983;**25**(1):56-59

[14] Myers MA, Rabin DU, Rowley MJ. Pancreatic islet cell cytoplasmic antibody in diabetes is represented by antibodies to islet cell antigen 512 and glutamic acid decarboxylase. Diabetes. 1995;**44**(11):1290-1295

[15] Petruzelkova L et al. The dynamic changes of zinc transporter 8 autoantibodies in Czech children from the onset of Type 1 diabetes mellitus. Diabetic Medicine. 2014;**31**(2):165-171

[16] Dunseath G et al. Bridging-type enzyme-linked immunoassay for zinc transporter 8 autoantibody measurements in adult patients with diabetes mellitus. Clinica Chimica Acta. 2015;**447**:90-95

[17] Chen S et al. Sensitive non-isotopic assays for autoantibodies to IA-2 and to a combination of both IA-2 and GAD65. Clinica Chimica Acta. 2005;**357**(1):74-83

[18] Brooking H et al. A sensitive non-isotopic assay for GAD65 autoantibodies. Clinica Chimica Acta. 2003;**331**(1-2):55-59

[19] Insel RA et al. Staging presymptomatic type 1 diabetes: A scientific statement of JDRF, the Endocrine Society, and the American Diabetes Association. Diabetes Care. 2015;**38**(10):1964-1974

[20] Yu L et al. Distinguishing persistent insulin autoantibodies with differential risk: Nonradioactive bivalent proinsulin/insulin autoantibody assay. Diabetes. 2012;**61**(1):179-186

[21] Yu L et al. Proinsulin/Insulin autoantibodies measured with electrochemiluminescent assay are the earliest indicator of prediabetic islet autoimmunity. Diabetes Care. 2013;**36**(8):2266-2270

[22] Miao D et al. GAD65 autoantibodies detected by electrochemiluminescence assay identify high risk for type 1 diabetes. Diabetes. 2013;**62**(12):4174-4178

[23] Miao D et al. Electrochemiluminescence assays for insulin and glutamic acid decarboxylase autoantibodies improve prediction of type 1 diabetes risk. Diabetes Technology & Therapeutics. 2015;**17**(2):119-127

[24] Yu L. Islet autoantibody detection by electrochemiluminescence (ECL) assay. Methods in Molecular Biology. 2016;**1433**:85-91

[25] Steck AK et al. ECL-IAA and ECL-GADA can identify high-risk single autoantibody-positive relatives in the TrialNet pathway to prevention study. Diabetes Technology & Therapeutics. 2016;**18**(7):410-414

[26] Palmer JP. Insulin autoantibodies: Their role in the pathogenesis of IDDM. Diabetes/Metabolism Reviews. 1987;**3**(4):1005-1015

[27] Baekkeskov S et al. Identification of the 64 K autoantigen in insulin-dependent diabetes as the GABA-synthesizing enzyme glutamic acid decarboxylase. Nature. 1990;**347**(6289):151-156

[28] Rabin DU et al. Cloning and expression of IDDM-specific human autoantigens. Diabetes. 1992;**41**(2):183-186

[29] Wenzlau JM et al. The cation efflux transporter ZnT8 (Slc30A8) is a major autoantigen in human type 1 diabetes. Proceedings of the National Academy of Sciences of the United States of America. 2007;**104**(43):17040-17045

[30] Schlosser M et al. Diabetes Antibody Standardization Program: Evaluation of assays for insulin autoantibodies. Diabetologia. 2010;**53**(12):2611-2620

[31] Torn C et al. Diabetes antibody standardization program: Evaluation of assays for autoantibodies to glutamic acid decarboxylase and islet antigen-2. Diabetologia. 2008;**51**(5): 846-852

[32] Bonifacio E et al. Harmonization of glutamic acid decarboxylase and islet antigen-2 autoantibody assays for national institute of diabetes and digestive and kidney diseases consortia. The Journal of Clinical Endocrinology and Metabolism. 2010;**95**(7):3360-3367

[33] Yu L et al. Early expression of antiinsulin autoantibodies of humans and the NOD mouse: Evidence for early determination of subsequent diabetes. Proceedings of the National Academy of Sciences of the United States of America. 2000;**97**(4):1701-1706

[34] Bingley PJ, Bonifacio E, Mueller PW. Diabetes Antibody Standardization Program: First assay proficiency evaluation. Diabetes. 2003;**52**(5):1128-1136

[35] Wenzlau JM et al. Novel antigens in type 1 diabetes: The importance of ZnT8. Current Diabetes Reports. 2009;**9**(2):105-112

[36] Wang J et al. Prevalence of autoantibody-negative diabetes is not rare at all ages and increases with older age and obesity. The Journal of Clinical Endocrinology and Metabolism. 2007;**92**(1):88-92

[37] Achenbach P et al. Mature high-affinity immune responses to (pro)insulin anticipate the autoimmune cascade that leads to type 1 diabetes. The Journal of Clinical Investigation. 2004;**114**(4):589-597

[38] Liu E, Eisenbarth GS. Accepting clocks that tell time poorly: Fluid-phase versus standard ELISA autoantibody assays. Clinical Immunology. 2007;**125**(2):120-126

[39] Babaya N et al. Murine high specificity/sensitivity competitive europium insulin autoantibody assay. Diabetes Technology & Therapeutics. 2009;**11**(4):227-233

[40] Haskins K, Atkinson M. Prediction of diabetes and response to therapy in individual animals: Are there lessons for man? Report on the JDF/Snow Mountain Meeting, 5-7 October 2000, Winter Park, CO, USA. Journal of Autoimmunity. 2001;**16**(1):15-19

[41] Vehik K et al. Development of autoantibodies in the TrialNet Natural History Study. Diabetes Care. 2011;**34**(9):1897-1901

[42] Barker JM et al. Autoantibody "subspecificity" in type 1 diabetes: Risk for organ-specific autoimmunity clusters in distinct groups. Diabetes Care. 2005;**28**(4):850-855

[43] Triolo TM et al. Additional autoimmune disease found in 33% of patients at type 1 diabetes onset. Diabetes Care. 2011;**34**(5):1211-1213

[44] de Graaff LC, Smit JW, Radder JK. Prevalence and clinical significance of organ-specific autoantibodies in type 1 diabetes mellitus. The Netherlands Journal of Medicine. 2007;**65**(7):235-247

[45] Norris JM et al. Risk of celiac disease autoimmunity and timing of gluten introduction in the diet of infants at increased risk of disease. JAMA. 2005;**293**(19):2343-2351

[46] Liu E et al. Risk of pediatric celiac disease according to HLA haplotype and country. The New England Journal of Medicine. 2014;**371**(1):42-49

[47] Gesualdo PD et al. Feasibility of screening for T1D and celiac disease in a pediatric clinic setting. Pediatric Diabetes. 2016;**17**(6):441-448

[48] Zhang B et al. A plasmonic chip for biomarker discovery and diagnosis of type 1 diabetes. Nature Medicine. 2014;**20**(8):948-953

[49] Tsai CT et al. Ultrasensitive Antibody Detection by Agglutination-PCR (ADAP). ACS Central Science. 2016;**2**(3):139-147

[50] Yim SW et al. Four-color alternating-laser excitation single-molecule fluorescence spectroscopy for next-generation biodetection assays. Clinical Chemistry. 2012;**58**(4):707-716

[51] Bale SS et al. A highly sensitive microsphere-based assay for early detection of Type I diabetes. Technology. 2014;**02**(03):200-205

[52] Ziegler AG et al. 3 screen ELISA for high-throughput detection of beta cell autoantibodies in capillary blood. Diabetes Technology & Therapeutics. 2016;**18**(11):687-693

[53] Zhao Z et al. A multiplex assay combining insulin, GAD, IA-2 and transglutaminase autoantibodies to facilitate screening for pre-type 1 diabetes and celiac disease. Journal of Immunological Methods. 2016;**430**:28-32